The
Diminished
Mind

One Family's Extraordinary Battle with Alzheimer's

The Jean Tyler Story
by Harry Anifantakis

Foreword by Jay M. Ellis, D.O.
Associate Professor of Neurology
University of Massachusetts Medical School

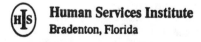
Human Services Institute
Bradenton, Florida

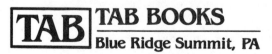
TAB BOOKS
Blue Ridge Summit, PA

FIRST EDITION
FIRST PRINTING

Produced by Book Creations, Inc.
Lyle Kenyon Engel, Founder

Library of Congress Cataloging-in-Publication Data

Tyler, Jean, 1933 –
　　The diminished mind : one family's extraordinary battle with
　Alzheimer's / the Jean Tyler story by Harry Anifantakis.
　　　p.　　cm.
　　ISBN 0-8306-3465-7
　　1. Tyler, Manley—Mental health.　2. Alzheimer's disease-
　-Patients—Massachusetts—Biography.　3. Mental health services-
　-Massachusetts.　I. Anifantakis, Harry.　II. Title.
　RC523.T95　1990
　362.1'96831—dc20　　　　　　　　　　　　　　90-35276
　　　　　　　　　　　　　　　　　　　　　　　　　　　CIP

TAB BOOKS offers software for sale. For information and a catalog, please contact TAB Software Department, Blue Ridge Summit, PA 17294-0850.

Questions regarding the content of this book should be addressed to:

Reader Inquiry Branch
TAB BOOKS
Blue Ridge Summit, PA 17294-0850

Acquisitions Editor: Kimberly Tabor
Book Design: Joanne M. Slike
Production: Katherine G. Brown
Typesetting: Terry W. Hite
Cover Design: Lori E. Schlosser
Cover Photograph: Susan M. Riley, Harrisonburg, VA

To the two greatest blessings
of my life—Laurie and Steven.

Jean Tyler

Acknowledgments

My heartfelt thanks to Laurie Rosin, Editorial Director at Book Creations. She saw the value of this book from the beginning and tirelessly worked to convince others to believe in it. Jean and I are indebted to her for her unwavering enthusiasm, professionalism, and skill, which triumphed over all obstacles in editing the difficult material in this true story. Thanks also to George and Marla Engel, Judy Stockmayer, and the rest of the staff at Book Creations.

I feel privileged to know the Tyler family. Getting to know Laurie and Art DelNegro, Steven and Belinda Tyler, and Jean's other relatives and friends has been deeply rewarding for me. Their openhearted honesty and encouragement were essential to making this book come alive. I am grateful for their trust and friendship.

Though I never met Manley Tyler, I feel I have come to know him through his family and friends. Much of this book portrays Manley when he was not himself. When he was well, he had a forceful personality that was balanced by the capacity to express love and gentleness. He was as complex as he was brilliant. Though he had frailties, as we all do, he never wavered from his passionate commitment to helping the underdog and encouraging those less fortunate than himself. He had the intellectual potential to be almost anything. It is a measure of the man that he chose to educate and nurture the minds of the young. I wish I could have known him personally.

Jean Tyler is a remarkable woman, but she would be the last to think so. Although she sought no personal recognition, she became a persuasive leader and activist on behalf of caregivers everywhere who humbly do a thankless job. I have tried to bring her multifaceted personality to life in this book. I see in her the best of our world: nonjudgmental love and earthy humor. I believe that love is always at the root of true heroism. She is an example of the unsung heroes around us, and I hope my words do her justice.

HARRY M. ANIFANTAKIS
CANAAN, NEW YORK

v

A Note from the Tyler Family

The decision to have this book written, subsequently allowing our family ordeal with Alzheimer's disease to become public knowledge, was extremely difficult. However, the need to inform more people of the daily reality of living with Alzheimer's and the plight of the caregivers overcame our initial and personal reluctance.

As you read our book, please remember that it has not been written because we are unique or special people, rather because *we are not*! There are millions of people who are at this moment suffering and struggling to deal with this dread disease. While their accounts may differ slightly from ours, their pain, frustration, and exhaustion are no less real. If, indeed, you are moved to tears, let the tears be for them.

My hope is that when you close the book and go about your life you will have a better understanding of what your neighbor may be suffering. Therefore, be more supportive, caring, and willing to help us in our fight against the debilitating disease of Alzheimer's.

JEAN TYLER

Foreword

Alzheimer's disease is a dreaded, horrible condition that affects many of our citizens, striking some younger individuals as well as a high percentage of the elderly. This illness strikes at the very core of our being, depriving the individual of the qualities that endeared them to all around them. There is little physical pain, disfigurement, or mutilation; thus, the community cannot see the suffering in a sense that would immediately invoke an appropriate caring response. Instead, the disease insidiously robs the victims of their unique thought processes, their insights, their judgment, their ability to learn new information—i.e., to form recent memories. Without these capabilities, the adult human regresses to an earlier, dependent life. The decline is slow and inexorable, but variable and thus unpredictable. The casual observer of such a person can scarcely note the failing; inescapably disparaging psychological explanations come forth. The victims are blamed for their illness. By the time a diagnosis is made, the individual has endured ruin in a physical, emotional, social, and financial sense.

Our brains are complex organs designed to take in information from our environment, sort out what is to be kept, tie that data into previously acquired data, and then cause the remaining brain to act on that input. Alzheimer's is a peculiar neurologic illness in which nerve cells in critical brain areas disappear and their vital association pathways are lost. The sensory input of living continues but is not stored, processed, or associated; the output becomes more and more limited. We can measure central nervous system function only by seeing the performance.

As a result of the loss of the patient's own faculties, other methods must develop to interpret and utilize the sensory input. The families of Alzheimer's victims have an increasingly important role in this realm. They must find ways to cope with increased responsibilities for managing the affairs of their dementing loved one. At the same time, they have to absorb the loss of a former source of strength. Frequently they themselves are bewildered by the problem in the early stages. Family members are critical of the ill person for "not trying hard enough." Only gradually does the harsh reality set in. Systematically, the support people come forward—amazingly at times—and take over functions of judgment, management of finances, decision making, remembering of necessary facts, and protection against emotional damage. This aspect, the caretaker role, has not received enough attention. Jean Tyler and her family exemplify the struggles that are occurring daily in this situation.

The devastation of the person by Alzheimer's has been recognized only in recent times. Before 1980, scant concern was shown for the victims and their courageous families. Through hard work, sensitivity, perseverance, and determination, Jean Tyler has done a great deal to change that circumstance in New England. At a time when she was enduring the torment of her beloved husband's illness, then his death, she used her seemingly tireless energy to help ensure that other families would not have to cope with Alzheimer's without emotional support, education, guidance, and wise advice. Almost invariably, I found myself referring one family after another to Jean as soon as I was certain of the diagnosis. My observation was that these people gained more from their contact with her than from any medical resource. She has aided more people by sharing her experience, wisdom, and concern than can be grasped.

Although Jean does not intend this book as a tribute to herself, she certainly deserves the rightful recognition for all that she has done. From this book may come the strength that can carry others through the ordeal Jean has managed so well for her family. Perhaps it will also spur legislative action to support Alzheimer's research and to make laws protecting the financial well-being of these caretaker families. No respite was ever available for Jean or her family. Surely a kinder, gentler nation that can produce the great technological and military organizational achievements of our country can create some better way to care for these dementing individuals. How a nation cares for its weaker members may well define its strengths.

From a neurological perspective, it seems that to solve the enigma of dementia, one will either have to stop the loss of the critical nerve cells or will have to re-create the pathways for synthesis and transmission of information. The challenge will require enormous research and interplay of multiple disciplines. Until that work comes to fruition, our society would do well to learn from experiences like Jean's to deal with the consequences of this illness.

DR. JAY MARK ELLIS
Pittsfield, Massachusetts

Part
I

1986

$\mathcal{D}$riving through the red and gold woods on this back road was an exhilarating experience for Jean Tyler. While on her way to work, she could relive moments from simpler, easier times and taste again the feeling of solid well-being she'd enjoyed most of her life. The sloping hills and distant mountain ridges, glowing with the beauty of early October in New England, had the same wordless power over her as they had had long ago. The earth alone seemed constant in her existence, for within the last few years, change had reshaped her life and the lives of the people around her.

Never far from her thoughts was the fact that she had lost Manley, her husband and soul mate. He had been lost for years now. He still lived—or his body did—in the Veterans Administration Hospital in Northampton, Massachusetts, but a disease called Alzheimer's had ruined his brain. As months stretched cruelly into years, Jean's loss had become a fact of daily life.

It wasn't a very long trip from her apartment across the Massachusetts border into Stanford, Vermont, where she worked on the advertising staff of a young corporation. She enjoyed the ride, especially since she had found a way through the back roads that was more scenic and less trafficked.

In the old days before Manley's illness she had rarely driven a car. Now her blue Subaru sedan was very important to her, providing one of the few ways she could be alone and undistracted by the many ongoing demands on her time. When she was troubled by something, she would often retreat into her car and take a long ride. Her thoughts and emotions had a chance to settle down again, away from the telephone and associations of the past that were everywhere around her at home.

All too quickly she arrived, parked the car, and walked to the corporation's main building. The morning air smelled of wet, freshly fallen autumn leaves. For a moment the aroma reminded her of other autumns, long past, and she had an urge to run beyond the building and kick through a pile of brown oak leaves. She smiled faintly to herself and entered the building.

As she passed through the front lobby, the receptionist signaled to her.

"You had a telephone call, Jean, from the hospital. They said you should contact them right away." The young woman handed Jean a slip of paper with the name Ruth Bateman and a phone number written on it.

"Thanks, Carol." She took it and walked to her office. Ruth was the head nurse in the wing of the hospital where Manley was cared for. Jean had become used to such messages, usually relating to the ups and downs of Manley's condition.

She called the hospital and was put on hold while the switchboard paged Ruth. The thought crossed Jean's mind, as it had hundreds of times before, that Manley had died. But in reality, Ruth's calls were usually requests for Jean's input in making decisions concerning Manley's treatment. She would say: "Come down when you have a chance, Jean. There's no rush."

This time it was different. Ruth's familiar voice had a flat quality to it.

"Hi, Jean. Things are not too good with Manley. In fact, they're very bad. I think you should come right away. It's hard to know for sure, but we feel he won't last out the day."

Jean sighed grimly. "Okay, Ruth. Thank you. I'll leave immediately." Sixteen months earlier she had gotten a similar message. Manley had almost died then, but his strong body had survived the pneumonia.

She called her daughter, Laurie, a high achiever with seemingly inexhaustible energy. She had just turned thirty, and besides being a wife and mother of two delightful girls, she did well at selling real estate.

Laurie answered the phone. "Brookfield Properties."

"I just got a call from the hospital. They told me to come right away."

"What did they say, Mom?"

"Ruth doesn't think Dad will last out the day. This looks like *it*."

"I'm coming with you, Mom. Art can take care of Kate and

Kara. Just give me an hour."

"I'll wait for you at the apartment."

"Are you okay?"

"Oh, sure," Jean answered automatically. Then with sarcasm, "Do I have a choice?"

Laurie laughed nervously. "I know. Just go home. I'll be there soon."

Jean hung up and sat very still for a moment. Although she had been preparing for years for Manley's death, she was confronted by deep confusion and ambivalence. At this point, although it was logically better that Manley die sooner than later, her immediate reaction was to save him at any cost. But save him for what? For fifteen years Alzheimer's disease had been working against Manley Tyler, confounding his mind in the beginning, robbing his ability to remember, blurring his sense of self, and finally reducing his mental capacity to that of an infant. Once he had been an educator of profound skill and dedication, giving his all to the immense challenge of nourishing and guiding young minds. But his athletic body, diminished to a shadow of what it had once been, was failing. It left his spirit no option but to move on.

By now Jean was a veteran of hospital life, but she had little experience with death. Her father's death from leukemia thirteen years before had been an entirely different situation because his mind hadn't been affected. He'd been perfectly lucid and able to communicate what was on his mind, what he wanted, right up to the end. She could do things for him and know he felt better, because he told her so.

Manley, on the other hand, could do no such thing. He couldn't talk, couldn't think; he barely reacted at all now. So Jean would do and do for him, yet never be certain that she had done the right things. Manley couldn't tell her. All his caregivers could do was guess about his needs. There had been times when he had become agitated, showing a remnant of his old, fierce temper, and the hospital staff were relatively sure that his acting out had been due to pain—his vertebrae were deteriorating. Giving him morphine helped that problem. But they could be sure about little else.

Jean's drive back to North Adams lacked the charm of her earlier ride to work. When she returned to her apartment, she made a phone call to her aunt Grace and uncle Jim. Like others, Grace and Jim had been of invaluable help and comfort through the often tumultuous times.

She checked the messages on her answering machine. The hos-

5

pital had called here before leaving a message for Jean at work. There was also a call from a woman seeking support for her family; her mother had been diagnosed to have Alzheimer's disease. Jean wrote down the name and number.

Laurie arrived shortly, and they left in her car. During the hour-long drive to Northampton they spoke of everyday events and even joked nervously, making the best of things moment by moment, as they had done for so long now. Jean noticed that despite the ominous summons, the world still was incredibly beautiful this morning.

Though her life had become progressively more complicated and difficult as the years passed, Jean had valiantly carried on, doing everything in her power to keep Manley as happy as possible. Their two children, Laurie and Steven, were adults now. Steven, younger than his sister by seven years, had spent much of his childhood and his entire adolescence influenced by the chaos of his father's illness. Under his mother's careful eye and with the help of relatives and family friends, he had survived. Now stationed in Panama, he held an important position in United States Air Force Intelligence.

We're still a family, Jean thought, looking proudly at her daughter. *And we're closer than ever.* She shook her head in wonderment. It was amazing how much suffering human beings could endure. She felt as if she had spent lifetimes in the hospital and at home, in rooms grown heavy with stubborn love, defying the disease, caring for a man once so splendid, as the vibrance of his mind and body emptied day by day for fifteen unstoppable years.

When Jean and Laurie walked into Manley's hospital room, his eyes were closed, and his upper body was propped up by pillows to ease his breathing. In the five and a half years he'd been in the hospital, this was his ninth battle with pneumonia. Natalie, a nurse's assistant, sat near the foot of Manley's bed. There was always someone with him these days. The staff that took care of him were remarkably thoughtful and compassionate. They genuinely liked Manley. Jean had blessed them in her mind many times. Over the years these nurses, assistants, and other health-care professionals had become an intimate extension of the family. Jean thought, *What a true hell this would be without Ruth, Natalie, and the others who care for Manley.*

She went to her husband and, reaching over the side railing, gently shook his shoulder. "Hi, Manley," she said cheerfully. "It's Jean, dear. How're you doing?"

His eyes opened, and he reacted, as usual, with a momentary glow of recognition in his eyes. She kissed him warmly on the cheek and mouth.

"Hi, Daddy," Laurie said from the other side of the bed. She squeezed his hand and, always on the alert for a glimmer of awareness, watched the blank stare on his face. She bent and touched his cheek, then kissed it. His eyes moved partway in her direction. "Hi, Dad," Laurie repeated, louder, with a smile. "Love you." His eyes closed wearily again.

But peacefully, Jean thought.

Laurie's eyes strayed to the bulge at Manley's stomach. Heavy bandaging beneath the sheet kept the food tube securely in position. The tube fed nutrients directly into his stomach. It had caused problems, including recurring infection. The smile slipped from Laurie's face.

Jean noticed and quipped, "Heck of a way to get a drink." This brought a less pained expression back to her daughter's face.

As she always did, Laurie started telling Manley what his granddaughters had been up to and other events within the family. Jean smiled. Laurie always had gossip for her father. It did not matter that he understood none of it, as long as he *might* feel the familial warmth of it, that he was loved, that he was a part of life.

No machines were attached to Manley—no respirators, monitors, or IV paraphernalia. The single food tube and periodic intramuscular injections of morphine were the only concessions to modern technology.

"Utilize everything to keep him as comfortable as possible," Jean had told the hospital staff. "I want him to suffer no pain. But he must be allowed to die." That was the only choice in this case, and knowing Manley, she knew that he would have agreed totally.

She stopped herself from dwelling on what might have been had he stayed healthy, yet she couldn't help but remember him with fascinated pleasure. Life with Manley Tyler had not been dull.

He'd been a tenacious man with a temper, strong opinions about everything, and the great imaginative impetus to explore life fully. In high school he had been a basketball star who had attracted the attention of young coeds. With his terrific looks and exceptional mind, the sky seemed the only limit. Manley was ambitious, fastidious, and organized. He burned with an absolute passion for music.

The pursuit of knowledge was the ideological engine that drove him. Although history was his favorite subject, he had voracious curiosity in every discipline. A flair for the dramatic and a charismatic presence helped him to capture the hearts and minds of all who knew him. He'd been a natural at teaching because he so loved to learn, and under his tutelage, students were inspired to feel the same love.

His style as a principal and teacher was that of an entertaining but stern disciplinarian, perhaps influenced by his military service during World War II. He upheld very definite, uncompromising standards for himself and his students, but everyone judged him to be consistent and fair. His main goal had always been that students should get the most out of their time in school. As with the majority of exceptional teachers, he gained excellent results and had devoted followers because he truly cared about each individual student.

Jean recalled a scene described by one of Manley's fellow teachers, Doug Moore. "Manley's amazing," Doug had told her. "I don't know how he does it. One day, at lunchtime, the school cafeteria was noisier than usual. It was pandemonium—hundreds of voices yammering away, shouts across the room, even an occasional flying object. All of a sudden the din quieted. I looked around to see why and noticed that Manley had just walked in. He has that kind of effect. He's not an ogre at all, but he gets real respect. And they *like* him, too."

Now Jean went into the adjacent room, which was a nurse's lounge equipped with chairs, a table, lockers, and the all-important coffee machine. Only half the time she spent in the hospital was at Manley's side. She had to move around, wander in and out, chat with whoever was there. Laurie, on the other hand, stayed by her father's bed most of the time and could maintain long monologues for Manley's benefit. Ordinarily Jean and Laurie would visit at different times. Jean often came with another relative or friend, and Laurie usually came with her husband, Art, and in earlier days, with little Kate and Kara.

Jean poured coffee into a Styrofoam cup and sat at her customary place, the chair closest to the door. This put her barely six feet from the foot of Manley's bed, beyond the doorway. She lit a cigarette and stared through the room's single window. Sunlight lit the beech tree in the parking lot, and a breeze stirred its bright, gold leaves.

What a tortuous road we've traveled, Manley. After a life

time's habit, she couldn't stop confiding her deepest thoughts to her husband. *A beautiful life until it took that cruel turn. Anyway, we had twenty glorious years.*

Ruth Bateman and Laurie walked in, interrupting Jean's reverie. The head nurse spoke gravely and calmly, in the manner of the friend she had become. "He's sinking fast now. We don't expect him to last much longer. Did you notice how cold his hands are? And the whiteness of his nails?" Jean and Laurie nodded. "Dr. Peters will be here soon. I just wanted to let you know so you can be prepared."

Laurie stared wordlessly, large tears rolling down her cheeks. Jean put an arm around her daughter and hugged her. *How hard to say good-bye.* After so many years she had no urge to weep, but something inside her clenched and hurt. *Why did this happen to a love as deep as ours, Manley? You are my truest friend.*

Ruth continued. "I can tell you honestly that I have rarely seen a person as lucky as Manley. You've minimized his suffering, and you both should feel good about that. The man really hasn't had a chance to feel lonely." This elicited weak but grateful smiles.

Jean and Laurie returned to the bedside and succumbed to an unusual silence, deep in their own thoughts, as they watched the still, frail body. Jean wondered what remained of her husband's consciousness. Could he think clearly at times, even now? How much of what they said did he comprehend? There were widely divergent medical opinions on that subject.

No one knew for sure what thoughts or feelings might be hidden behind a face that had become more masklike with each bewildering year. Jean once said, "You can tell a lot from Manley's eyes: When he is his old self, his eyes show it, even if his intelligence has been drastically reduced. But at other times his eyes get a dead look to them, and you know he's not . . . there. *That's* not Manley."

Laurie and Steven had been very close with their father. Manley's skill and understanding of children had made for an exceptionally rich and healthy homelife. For Laurie the onset of Manley's illness had come when her adult life was just beginning, depriving her of a sense of real freedom at the time when it should have been at its height. Still, she fell in love, married Art, a gentle bear of a man, and started a family of her own, though her attentions were spread thin at times.

Steven had been a mere eight years old when his father's personality had begun to change. That early symptom was particularly confusing for Steven. As he grew through the crucial times of puberty and adolescence, he experienced the gradual disappearance of his father and friend, while, perversely, Manley's physical presence remained unchanged. Jean's constant worry was that Steven might be emotionally scarred for life.

She had found herself drawing on strength she barely knew she had and became the anchor for the family's adjustment. The weight of responsibility for emotional as well as financial support fell to her, but she and her children had pulled together. It was a monumental task, made that much more difficult because Manley was young and strong. Rarely did Alzheimer's disease afflict people before old age, much less at age forty-two, when Manley's earliest symptoms appeared. Jean had been forced to make very difficult decisions. To keep Manley at home as long as possible was damaging to Steven, but her first thought was for her husband's welfare.

Just before noon Dr. Peters, Manley's primary physician, came in to examine his patient. Jean and Laurie waited for him in the nurse's lounge. When he joined them, his face was impassive.

"I can't see how it can be much longer," he said plainly. "He's fading. We've seen him like this a few times, of course, but from the signs I'd be surprised if he lasts more than another hour or two. He's in no pain. It's just a matter of time."

An hour passed. Then another. Jean notified Steven, using a telephone on the first floor to call the International Red Cross. This was the quickest way to reach someone in the armed services and stationed out of the country. The Red Cross would relay the message, and Steven would call her back at the hospital. It was certain that Steven wouldn't see his father alive again, but he would have to come home anyway.

Late in the afternoon Aunt Grace and Uncle Jim arrived. Grace held Manley's limp hand.

"Hey, handsome. How are you, Son? Are these women taking good care of you?" No doom and gloom for Grace. "It's Grace, dear. Jim and Grace. Yes, we're back. Can't keep us away."

Jim stood close by, staring stoically, not saying much. Hospitals were not his favorite place, and it was very difficult for him to watch Manley as he was now.

They all took turns standing by Manley's bed. Each had a special way with him, talking about anything that came to mind in the faint hope that he might be aware of a friendly voice. Otherwise they sat in the lounge and talked quietly and drank coffee or juice. Aunt Grace eased the passage of time with current gossip. Jean smoked more than usual, but she didn't care. During her turn at the bedside, she mentioned that Steven would be coming. Though she knew that Steven would arrive too late, she stroked Manley's head and asked in her usual sunny way, "Won't it be nice to see Steven again, hon? And Belinda will be coming, too. Remember Steven's new wife? I really like that girl."

Laurie contributed to her relatives' conversation when she wasn't drifting in her own thoughts. Throughout the years of her father's illness she felt that she hadn't sacrificed as much or suffered as terribly as her mother and brother had. It bothered her deeply that she'd had to move out of her parents' house when she married Art, abandoning Jean and Steven to cope alone. Yet she truly had shared a great deal of the burden, as had Art: Before Manley was hospitalized, Laurie had taken him to her home often, to give her mother much needed breaks. With two young daughters to care for, Laurie did what she could, but to her it seemed pitifully inadequate.

She felt doubly bad about Steven because her own childhood and adolescence had been extraordinarily happy and full. She had a banquet of memories to feast from, with a father who genuinely enjoyed spending all his spare time with his children. With sweet sadness she remembered those innocent days, as distant now as a vintage fairy tale: enacting countless games and fantasies, trekking off to woods and fields, hiking, swimming, picnicking, taking car trips, singing in the car.

Manley had the childlike ability to create an adventure from the smallest opportunity. Once, when Laurie was thirteen, she had gone swimming with her father to Dobb's Pond just before dusk. It was really not much of a pond, and she had been less than enthusiastic, but Manley had talked her into it in his usual irresistible way. When they got there he had wanted to swim, but she had resisted. He splashed about, urging Laurie to join him. When she finally did enter the chilly water, the bottom muck sucked at her feet. She wondered why they were there, where no one ever swam. But in no time she was enjoying herself. Back and forth they swam in the murky water and the fading light, Manley's strong, lean body gliding effortlessly beside her as he joked with her. Now, seventeen years later, she found herself treasuring these things about her father that she had carelessly taken for granted as a youth.

At five o'clock another assistant, named Mike, replaced Natalie at the foot of Manley's bed. The tall, good-natured youth was another of Jean's favorites at the hospital. After carefully checking on Manley and tending to his needs, he greeted everyone cheerily. Laurie's mood improved. She always felt better when Mike was around.

Manley's breathing, though shallow and irregular, continued uninterrupted. He seemed comfortable, which was always Jean's top priority. Every few hours he had another shot of morphine to deaden the pain from his deteriorating spine.

During one of Laurie's times with Manley she paused in the flow of stories about her children and said, "Daddy, if you can hear me, squeeze my hand." She gave his hand a gentle squeeze.

A few minutes later she re-joined the others in the lounge. "Mom," she whispered. "I asked Dad to squeeze my hand if he could hear me, and he did! I swear he did. I mean, I was squeezing his hand, too, so I'm not sure what it means, but still . . ."

Aunt Grace, after hearing this, went quietly in to Manley. When she returned she said to Jean, "Laurie's right. I think he's stronger. He squeezed my hand, too."

Jean checked on him, and he did seem more alive somehow. She could tell from the shine in his eyes.

There was no change into the evening. They could do nothing but wait. At about ten o'clock Mike looked in on them. "Jean, you haven't eaten all day, have you? You have to get some food."

She smiled at the young man who took such good care of her husband. "Don't start now, Mike. I'm not hungry. I've been drinking plenty of your coffee."

Mike looked at Laurie. "When did you guys eat last?"

Laurie thought for a moment. "Breakfast, I guess."

"This youngster's right," Grace said. "It's time we got some nourishment. I, for one, am starved."

Mike looked over at Uncle Jim, who smiled and rolled his eyes with a shrug. "C'mon now," Mike urged. "You're going to get some dinner if Jim and I have to carry you out. Don't worry about Manley. Tell me where you're going to be, and I'll let you know immediately if there's any change. No arguments."

Jean finally relented. "Okay, okay, if you're all going to gang up on me . . . I guess I could eat something."

"We'll go to Friendly's Restaurant down the street," Jim told Mike as he rose from his chair.

Everyone was hungry. Even Jean ate half a sandwich. No call came from Mike.

When they returned to the hospital, Ruth, Mike, and a new

12

doctor were gathered around Manley. Mike joined the family in the nurse's lounge. "Manley's definitely doing better for some reason," he reported. "When Ruth noticed, she called the doctor."

The head nurse came in, followed by the doctor, a friendly looking, smallish man Jean had seen but never met. "I'm Dr. Elliot," he said. "Well, it seems he's really perked up. All his vital signs are accelerating. It's unusual. I don't honestly know what to make of it. This was unexpected, but now he's holding on with a vengeance."

"We're sure he'll last the night now," added Ruth. "He seems to be fighting."

"Why? Why now?" Jean asked.

"It's hard to say," the doctor answered. "It's puzzling."

They all waited for another forty-five minutes before deciding they should go home for the night. Mike assured Jean that she would be notified if anything significant happened, no matter what time it was. They left just before midnight.

At 7:15 A.M. the telephone rang next to Jean's bed. She picked it up and came instantly awake when she heard her son's voice.

"Steven? What time? . . ." She glanced at the clock beside her.

"Hi, Mom. How's Dad?"

"Bad, Steven. He's not expected to live much longer. They didn't expect him to make it through yesterday. It was hour by hour. He rallied last night, but no one knows how much longer he can hang on. I figured I'd better let you know."

"Thanks, Mom." He was silent for a moment. Then, "How are *you* doing? Are you handling it okay?"

"Oh, well. It's no picnic, but I'm all right. Yes. Laurie and I are hanging in here." She paused and gathered her thoughts. Then, "Steven, I need you here. I need you so badly. We've come full circle. I can't make it without you now."

Over the phone she could sense that Steven was making a decision. "I'm going to leave right away," he said. "I'll talk to my C.O. I'm not sure when the flights are. You'll be at the hospital?"

"Yes." She gave him the number. "If Dad's still hanging on, we'll be back home at midnight, I guess."

"I'll call you tonight at midnight and let you know what we're doing. I'm not sure how soon I can leave."

When Steven hung up he called his commanding officer and

explained the situation. After getting permission to leave immediately, Steven phoned Belinda, who packed a suitcase.

Steven drove home quickly, parked the car, and left the motor running. While Belinda put her things in the car, he threw some clothes into a suitcase, locked the house, and in minutes they were speeding for the airport. They just made the flight.

The slow C-130 transport crept northward from Panama City. The morning's rush gave way to a drawn-out wait. In the quiet moments Steven thought about his parents. It was difficult for him to comprehend what the past fifteen years had been like for his mother or his father. To him those years were now a merciful blur, a smoky netherworld of memories, of vague guilt, of suppressed anger, and of trying to shoulder some of the responsibility that his mother carried. Looking back now as an adult, he was amazed that his mother and sister were as mentally healthy as they were. The grim inevitability of his father's deterioration had built itself around his own young mind like a thickening wall, causing him to lose interest in school and social life.

Some time after his father had finally been placed in the care of professionals, the song "I Made It Through the Rain" by Barry Manilow was popular on the radio. For Steven it symbolized the rite of passage they had all endured. Once, when he had been home on furlough, he'd called Jean's attention to it. "This song's for you, Mom," he told her. "It's for you. You really did make it through the rain."

She had looked fondly at her sturdy nineteen-year-old son, who had caused her such worry. "It's been hard, hasn't it, Steven? Do you think you're all right?"

"I'm fine, Mom. I can handle it."

"I worry about you. I don't want you crippled for the rest of your life. You're just an innocent victim—"

"We all are," he interrupted. He hated being singled out just because he was the youngest. They all had suffered.

"I guess you're right," Jean replied. "But you're the most vulnerable. And you don't seem to have a direction."

"I don't want to talk about it," he had said. The subject was closed. He wanted to deal with it on his own. He would need time, but he knew he'd be okay. "Anyway, Mom," he'd concluded, "this song's for you."

In the ensuing years the air force had proved to be a real opportunity for Steven. The service had tested him for aptitude, and his scores in language and cryptology proved to be the highest first-time results the administrators had ever seen. They soon set him on a course of intensive education, grooming him for a position in Air Force Intelligence. He had more than fulfilled their hopes for him.

As a solid career unfolded, he had met and fallen in love with Belinda in her hometown of San Angelo, Texas. She had a happy disposition and wisdom that belied her nineteen years. After a short time they were married.

At the wedding reception Steven had asked the disk jockey if he had the recording "I Made It Through the Rain." When it was played he took his mother's hand and led her onto the dance floor. "Remember this song?" he had asked her.

"I sure do."

"Well, now *I've* finally made it through the rain."

"You certainly have. It makes me feel good." Jean laughed. "There were times when I wondered. . . ."

"I know." He grinned. "But I'm fine now. So this time the song's for me."

That morning at the hospital Dr. Peters was on duty. He told Jean, "I don't know where Manley's getting the strength, but he's showing readings he hasn't had for a long time. Respiration, blood pressure, heart rate—they're all going full tilt. It doesn't make sense."

Ruth Bateman, who seemed to know Manley's moods and phases better than anyone, confided to Jean, "He's fighting with everything he's got to stay alive. I know he is. Supposedly he has no mind and therefore no will. But you can't tell me he isn't in there fighting. We gave him something to calm him down. And the morphine injections are continuing, but it's as if he doesn't want to be calm. He's quite a guy."

"Yesterday I told him that Steven is coming home to see him," Jean told the head nurse. "Do you think that has anything to do with it?"

"You mean, did he hear you and understand?" Ruth's steady expression wavered, and she thought for a moment. "Supposedly that's not possible. But . . . who really knows?"

Steven and Belinda continued their long day of traveling. In the afternoon their plane landed in Charleston, South Carolina, where they waited for a commercial flight to take them to Hartford, Connecticut, with a stopover in Washington, D.C. After they took off again, a new passenger was sitting next to Steven. They began to converse and discovered an amazing coincidence: Not only were they both deplaning in Hartford, they were both headed for North Adams, Massachusetts. Steven told the man about his father and the reason for their trip. The fellow offered to give Steven and Belinda a ride after they arrived in Hartford. He had a taxi waiting to take him all the way to North Adams. Steven gratefully accepted.

Jean and Laurie waited. Staff members were shaking their heads, incredulous at the radical change in Manley's condition. Grace and Jim came again later in the day. It was always good to have them around. There was a different kind of expectancy now, which continued unabated. Manley Tyler's metabolism raced like an engine at full throttle.

Steven is coming home, Jean thought with mounting excitement. So much of Manley was in Steven: his temperament, idealism, honesty, even his mannerisms. Laurie had inherited Manley's stoic integrity, his perfectionism, and his fierce drive. Despite all that had happened, Jean Tyler felt she was a lucky woman. She had two fine, noble children.

The nurses and other staff were watching Manley very closely, feeling he was in an unpredictable state. A nurse Jean had not met before came regularly and anointed Manley's eyes with something. "To keep them moist," she told Jean. "He's losing liquids because he's so pumped up."

Jean was more easily persuaded to go out for something to eat this evening, but she still made sure the staff on duty knew where the family was going to be. They all decided to go home earlier than before because the nurses assured them that Manley was "out of danger" for the time being. They promised that they would call Jean immediately if something serious happened. After saying good night in the parking lot, they all rode wearily home.

Jean hadn't been in her apartment twenty minutes when there was a turn of a key in her front-door lock, accompanied by knocking. In walked Steven and Belinda.

"I knew I was going to talk to you at midnight," Jean said amid embraces, "but I had no idea it would be in *person.* You move fast!"

In the excitement of their reunion, fatigue was forgotten, and they talked for hours. None of them slept much that night.

The first thing Jean did on awakening was to call the hospital to check on Manley. He seemed to be continuing the same as he had been, fighting to hang on. Jean called again before they left for Northampton. Laurie joined them, and they all went in one car, stopping along the way to eat a quick breakfast. They reached the hospital around ten o'clock.

Steven went in alone to see his father. Jean noticed that he prepared himself before he walked through the door, as he always had these past years: He straightened up to his full height, took a steadying breath, then went in, closing the door behind him.

It hurt to see his father like this. Manley had always been vigorous and athletic, even in the early years of the disease. Steven remembered his father's compassionate presence and the warmth of his laughter—two reasons why all kinds of people seemed to like Manley so much. The older Steven got, the more he understood how special his father had been. He hadn't been the type to fall into the easy groove of a glorified male ego. And now here he lay, so small, so frail. Steven took up his father's hands, then leaned down and gave him a hug around the neck. "Hi, Dad. Good to see you, old buddy!"

The family had told him all about how his father seemed to be fighting to hang on. More than ever Steven believed in the spirit. For a moment he was at a loss. What could he say? *I'm sorry you have to die. I'm sorry you've had to live this way for so long.* How much, if anything, would his father understand? His moment of doubt fled when he looked into those eyes he knew so well.

"Belinda and I just got in at midnight last night, Dad. It was quite a trip. I think we set some kind of record getting here."

What was it like to be imprisoned behind those eyes, which looked out from sunken hollows?

"Dad, I love you. We all love you. Don't you worry about us. We're doing fine. I'm fine, and so is Belinda. Laurie and Art are doing great, as always. The kids, too. And Mom is good, real good. She'll be fine. You don't have to worry about us at all." He pulled up a chair and sat close, holding his father's hands in both of his. "I don't know what to say. I realize you can't talk. But I believe you know what's going on. Please don't feel bad about all this. We've had a wonderful life together. I'll never forget. Never. You're the best father anyone could have.

"Sure, it was tough for me at times. I was young. I had a lot of anger, a lot of confusion. But I want you to know I'm fine now. Really, I am. I know you care about that. You always cared so much. . . ."

17

Steven barely noticed his own tears as he talked. He had to make certain he said everything. This was for real. He wanted to make certain that his father had no doubts, no regrets, no guilt. Manley had always been such an aware man, so somewhere in his damaged mind he must have realized the hardship on his family. Steven had to set that mind at peace.

"I'm sorry for anything I ever did that hurt you or frustrated you, Dad. I never meant to hurt you. And I know you never meant to hurt me. This damned disease was just a disease. It had nothing to do with you. So don't regret anything. Please. Everyone understands completely.

"I'm gonna miss you, Dad. We all are. But don't suffer any more. It's okay to go now. You'll always be with us. Always. Absolutely. You're the best. Do you think I could ever forget what a wonderful friend you are? The suffering is over now. You don't have to stay if you don't want to. I'll take care of everything here. I believe something much better is in store for you after this."

Manley's eyes, bright with moisture, watched his son, and Steven gazed back with wonderment. "Wherever you're going from here, I'd go now, Dad. It's all right to let go. No one could be more loved than you, Dad."

While Steven was with Manley, a nurse walked in. Taking in the scene, she turned and left quickly but went immediately to Jean and the others.

"I went in by mistake," she told them. "What I saw amazed me. Manley's eyes had been so dry all day and night, I had been trying to keep them lubricated. He was so dehydrated, there was no moisture in his eyes. Well, just now tears were rolling down his face. It's hard to understand. Your son was talking to him quietly, and Manley just stared back with those tearful eyes."

Steven finally came out after about half an hour. He re-joined his family in the nurse's lounge and poured himself a cup of coffee. He studied his mother carefully. He felt more peaceful than he had in years. He wanted her to feel that way, too. "Is everything all right out here? How are you doing, Mom?"

She looked at him with a smile. "I feel a lot better now that you're here." She didn't ask the questions that went through her mind but contented herself by just watching her son.

As soon as Steven had re-joined the others in the lounge, Ruth

18

Bateman went in to check on Manley. Afterward the head nurse took Jean aside, putting her arm around her in a sisterly way. "It's begun now. Everything is slowing down."

"His metabolism is slowing?"

"Yes. Everything's starting to calm down. Don't ask me how, but I can tell you he's giving in. He's ready to go."

Jean looked at her, incredulous.

Ruth went on. "The only thing I can say is that it was the kid, Jean. It's got to be Steven. Manley *was* waiting for him. What else could it be? It's only been minutes since Steven left his side, and now Manley's whole metabolic rate has slowed to where it was a couple days ago. He's saying it's all right now. He's giving himself permission to die."

All day long they waited. Laurie, Steven, and Belinda caught up on each other's life. Laurie explained that Art was taking care of Kate and Kara. She wanted their father instead of a babysitter to be with them at this time. They were only six and three, but they were precocious, and they loved their grandpa.

Steven occasionally wandered around the hospital, looking for people he had come to know when he used to visit often. One of his favorites, a funny old man who had been a patient, had since died, but Steven managed to find others.

That's his way of dealing with it, Jean thought.

Later Laurie joined her brother on a tour of the hospital. They stopped at an exercise room, and both got on stationary bicycles and raced as if they were really moving. A baseball game was on a television against the wall, and Steven, a talented pitcher who had played semipro ball, became engrossed in it. Laurie tried to watch. In the old days she had been an avid Red Sox fan along with her father, but without him to watch with, she had lost interest in the game.

The day passed, and as night drew on they all gathered around Manley. There wasn't much talk anymore. A television droned nearby; there were the evening sounds of a hospital getting settled for the night. Laurie and Steven were on both sides of their father, each leaning their heads against his and stroking him softly. Jean held his hand, with Belinda close by. Ruth and Natalie and another nurse stayed near.

Thus did Manley Tyler finally come to rest. He drifted deeper into sleep, and his breathing quietly ceased. It was over.

For a long time they stayed around him, wet eyed, caught in a spell that an extraordinary moment casts on people. A man's suffering had ended. These staff members, who had grown to love this patient over the years, and the family, who held all the precious memories, turned to each other and embraced. In this lucid moment they glimpsed the truth in each other and openly shared the love they felt so deeply.

Slowly they disengaged themselves. The family and hospital staff said their final good-byes to each other. And to Manley.

Jean and Laurie led the way to the car. Steven automatically took the driver's seat, as he always did. His father was here. He was sure of it. *You're here, aren't you, Dad?* he thought. He felt like making a gesture. He wanted to laugh in the face of despair.

There were a few loose audio cassettes lying around the car. His eyes picked out one by Barry Manilow. It contained "I Made It Through the Rain."

He thought of the countless times they had all sung together as the family car barreled along, with his father's strong baritone booming out unabashedly. He looked behind him at his mother. "This would be appropriate, wouldn't it?" he asked, waving the cassette tape. She didn't answer. Propriety didn't seem to matter just now.

He put the cassette into the car's tape player and found the song. He turned up the volume and reached behind him to find his mother's hand. "This time it's for Dad," he said, and began to sing.

His voice grew stronger, and they all joined in. Laurie and Belinda reached out and held hands, too, forming a complete circle.

Tearfully but joyfully they sang, releasing something, celebrating something. Jean squeezed hard on the hands she held, feeling lightened by a powerful energy they shared. She felt a part of something timeless.

If anyone had been watching in that hospital parking lot so late on that October night, they would not have believed that these people had just lost a loved one. They appeared to be a car full of friends singing their heads off, but the voices formed a strange emotional pitch of sorrow and joy. They drowned out Barry Manilow's voice: "We made it through the rain. . . ."

CHAPTER 2

Spring
1971

*I*t was minutes before three o'clock, the end of the school day. Manley Tyler, principal of Clarksburg Elementary School, in a small rural community in western Massachusetts, palmed the worn basketball after catching his own rebound off the backboard. He pivoted and shot again with a grace that defied his inner gnawing despair; he was still a natural athlete at forty-two years of age, still a man with an unmistakable aura of self-mastery. The ball arced and flipped the net cleanly as it flew through the hoop.

Fear. He was not used to its strength-sapping force. Feeling queasy, Manley did not shoot the basketball again but walked away with it. He took his suit jacket from a chair as he left the gym and walked shakily upstairs.

The three o'clock bell rang like an echoing jeer through the hallway. Seconds later throngs of school children exploded from classrooms around him. Seeing him, the students slowed their exodus to an orderly but urgent walk to the front entrance. He could manage only weak smiles in response to their cheerful greetings. The piping voices seemed far away, and he felt out of harmony with the school, insulated in a wilderness of dissolving dreams like a condemned man among the living.

He turned the corner and saw teachers coming out of their classrooms, chatting across the hall as they, too, prepared to leave. Manley shook his head in disapproval. During his years as a teacher he rarely left school before five-thirty. It became customary for students, parents, and community members to find him in his classroom after hours. They would talk more freely than they ever did at monthly Parent-Teacher Group meetings. The impromptu discussions were often of crucial value to families and had added immeasurably to Manley's stature as a teacher and civic leader.

All his life he'd striven to be the best educator possible. He had acquired a reputation as a teacher who could handle the toughest problems with unerring instinct while also inspiring the genuine affection of his students. He made it his business to know each youngster. Despite his strict classroom discipline and stringent demands, Manley's students realized that he cared deeply for them and always treated them fairly. He was too dedicated to the future to sacrifice the quality of their education through shortcuts and laziness.

Manley Tyler was considered brilliant and articulate, with an undeniable presence that made people take notice wherever he was, whatever he was doing, including coaching sports for the YMCA, Little League, and church teams, or singing publicly on radio programs, at fund-raisers, and in local theater productions.

That was why, in 1969, he was offered the post of head administrator for kindergarten through eighth grade of the Clarksburg school system: He had earned the honor. Manley couldn't resist the promotion and pay increase, so he accepted and in that first year earned the school committee's praise for tightening the operation of the two schools under his jurisdiction.

But not long after he had been wooed into becoming principal, he'd suspected it was a mistake. He felt out of place as an administrator, too removed from the lifeblood of a school. Now, two years later, things were coming apart. The job was a burden, a muddle of overwhelming details that frustrated his exacting sense of orderliness. He seemed to have lost touch with the teachers, who, he thought, were running amok and pointing fingers at him.

Even the administrative staff and the committee members showed increasing irritation and gave him strange looks. Everyone seemed to take sides against him lately, insisting that he had said or done things he hadn't, as if conspiring to confound him. Increasingly, he lost his patience and showed his anger. Never in his life had things felt so odd, so out of control.

Now Manley escaped into his office. As he put the basketball away in his closet he saw himself in the mirror. His immaculate white shirt, elegantly knotted tie, and impeccable tweed suit neatly hid the disheveled wreck he was inside. The strong features of his handsome face belied his inner turmoil.

A year ago he had tried to resign as principal and return to teaching, but chagrined school-committee members had talked him out of it. He stayed on for another year, but now there were times he just didn't care about the job. That disturbed him most of all. He had always cared before.

He didn't feel like himself and had been examined by his family doctor, Bill Everett, to determine if he had a physical problem. But Manley proved to be in excellent health.

Manley wondered about himself. As confident and knowing as he'd always felt as a teacher, he couldn't understand why he'd suffered so much trouble being principal. It was as if the intuitive skills he once used with such a sure hand had mysteriously vanished. Being with kids always gave him a special satisfaction, and he missed the joy and intimacy of being right in the caldron of learning, the classroom. He had always identified with children. They were his deepest enjoyment, and he honored their honesty and directness. It was adults who did their best to ruin a perfectly good world.

All those teachers against me, Manley thought angrily, *siding with that foolish Bruce Walsh!*

He knew it had been a mistake to deal so rashly with the eighth-graders' young teacher. Manley had tried to be patient, but in his opinion the twenty-four-year-old Walsh wasn't serious about the needs of the children. He was bold and strong willed, and when he ignored Manley's criticism and advice, it had made Manley so furious that he tried to deny tenure to the young man.

Then, two weeks before, in early April, Bruce Walsh had called a special meeting of the school committee and brought all the Clarksburg Elementary teachers with him to dispute Manley's evaluation. Manley had tried to explain his reasoning, but it had been such a tense moment he'd done a poor job. He knew what he had meant to say, but his words had had no effect on his listeners. The three-man committee had sided with Walsh. Never had Manley felt so humiliated.

What is happening to me? he wondered. *Why have I lost control?*

He wrenched himself away from the mirror and stared out the window. Whatever the reason for this hell he found himself in, it had no end. He wasn't doing his job properly, and he couldn't abide that.

His course of action became suddenly clear and unavoidable. He reached a decision. Unbearable waves of emotion welled up and burned his eyes as he prepared a letter of resignation. After wiping away the tears with his handkerchief, he fled into the corridor. He was seeking distraction, but the agony followed him. Tonight was the monthly meeting of the school committee, when he would make his announcement.

What will I do to earn a living when I'm not here anymore?

Jean Oldham Tyler was in her kitchen cooking dinner. The aroma of the cherry pie baking in the oven filled the house as she prepared beef stroganoff on the electric stove. Buttercup and Daisy, the two cats, were sitting in the middle of the room, watching her. Babe, the big black dog, lay under the table in the dining nook, while Buttons, the Tylers' little dog, sat alertly near the side door where she could be the first to greet eight-year-old Steven.

It was almost four-thirty. Manley usually did not get home till almost six, but Jean didn't mind. He took his job very seriously, and as a principal, he continued the habit, which he'd begun as a teacher, of staying into the late afternoon. As a result, the sound of the car pulling into their driveway surprised her.

Through the window Jean saw Manley's brown Ford LTD roll to a stop. She walked outside to greet him, but he remained behind the wheel, very still, as if deep in thought.

"Are you going to get out and give me a kiss," she called, grinning, "or are you staying in the car?"

Still seated, he turned to her, and a wistful smile grew on his face.

"You're home earlier than usual," she said, walking to the car.

"I am? Oh. There's a school-board meeting tonight."

"I forgot. Are you hungry?"

"No," he said absently.

She frowned. He was always hungry. "You don't feel sick, do you?"

"No. Why?"

"You seem preoccupied. Have a hard day at work?"

"Yes." He got out of the car slowly, forgetting his briefcase on the seat. Jean reached in for it, then followed him into the kitchen. Over his shoulder he said, "I'm a little tired."

The dogs and Daisy greeted him, and he stooped to pet them. After a minute Manley poured himself a glass of water and drank slowly, leaning against the counter.

He looks exhausted, Jean thought. Usually after work he was full of fun, wisecracking about the day's events. She handed him the briefcase. "Why don't you take a nap? I'll wake you when it's time for dinner."

"Maybe I will," he said without conviction.

He walked into the hallway, hung his coat in the closet, then went into the den. She heard the creak of the rocking chair as he sat down.

When she looked in on him a minute later, he had turned the chair so he could stare out the window to the open field behind the house. Daisy sat purring in his lap. The dogs were at his feet.

"Anything wrong, dear?" she asked.

"Just thinking."

"About your job?" Jean moved behind him and massaged his shoulders and neck. His face showed strain, but at her touch he closed his eyes and seemed to relax. "Can I get you anything? A cup of coffee?"

"No, thanks."

"So what happened today?" she asked. He always shared his feelings with her.

"The usual. Nothing special."

"More trouble with Bruce Walsh?"

He nodded.

"Well, just forget about him for now. He'll learn."

"Yes."

She moved around the chair to look at Manley. His clear green eyes held none of their accustomed humor. Instead there was a searching quality that discomfited her.

"You're as beautiful as the day I met you, Jean. I'm a lucky man."

She went behind his chair again and hugged him around the neck. "And I'm an incredibly lucky woman," she said into his ear. "I couldn't be happier."

He kissed one of her arms and softly said, "I love you, Jean. The one central fact in my life is that I love you."

"Oh, Manley . . ."

She disengaged her arms and maneuvered herself into his lap, displacing Daisy. The fatigue seemed to leave him. The need in his kisses made her tremble. She leaned back to look at him.

"Feeling better, now?" she asked cheerfully.

A smile broke out on his face. "What do you think? Your kisses are the cure for any ailment *I'll* ever have."

She kissed him once more for good measure, then rose and mimed a waitress with pen poised on an imaginary pad and affected a no-nonsense tone. "You *must* be hungry. Let me get you something. What'll it be?"

He laughed. "Okay, okay. I'll have a coffee with cream, please."

"Coming right up, sir."

As she was pouring coffee for him their fifteen-year-old daughter, Laurie, came through the side door, carrying books and a large shoulder bag. Her dark hair flowed down her back, and her striking blue eyes, which she'd inherited from her mother, sparkled.

"Hi, Mom," she said and kissed her mother.

The dogs came running from the den, and Laurie deposited her books on the table and hugged the pets.

"Where's Dad?"

"In the den."

Jean brought Manley his coffee and a dish of home-baked cookies, just in case he wanted a snack. Laurie came in behind her with a glass of milk.

"Hi, Daddy." She kissed him on the cheek.

"Hi, Pumpkin." Daisy was back in Manley's lap, and Laurie patted the cat on the head.

Watching them, Jean smiled with contentment. Her life had turned out pretty much the way she'd envisioned it: She'd fallen in love with the finest man she could imagine, they had raised two healthy kids, and life had gotten richer as Laurie and Steven grew into full-fledged people. Not everybody was that lucky.

The smooth running of the family and home was her responsibility, and her job was an easy one. She and Manley were coproviders for the welfare and harmony of the family, and there was never much discord in the household. She had found her life's companion while only in her midteens and had grown to adulthood thoroughly enmeshed with her man. . . .

When Manley first appeared in Jean's life she was only fifteen years old and preoccupied with Jimmy Vitalla, a bold, attractive boy who played drums in a band. They'd been going steady for over a year, but the relationship seemed to be ending. Jean paid Manley very little attention, although he was obviously attracted to her. She knew him as the older boy who always managed to sit behind her in physics class. She had heard he'd been in the military and was finishing an interrupted high-school education. Although Manley had tried often to talk to her, Jean wasn't interested. She was accustomed to being approached by boys and knew how to rebuff them gently.

In fact, Jean's girlfriends were more impressed with Manley

than she was. He had talent, athletic prowess, a reputation for academic achievement, and good looks. When he and his friends walked by in the school hallway, the girls would whisper, "Isn't he gorgeous?" or "His name is *Manley*. Isn't that perfect?"

Jean, still under Jimmy's romantic spell, thought her friends were being silly, although she couldn't deny that there was something special about Manley Tyler.

One day the physics teacher was late in arriving, and the students waited in the hall for him. Manley said hello to Jean and asked her about herself. For once she welcomed his conversation because there was nothing else to do. His manner was so friendly that she enjoyed his attention. For the first time she realized how strikingly good-looking he was, with high cheekbones and curly dark hair. His lively green eyes had a warmth that made her feel good.

The more they talked, the more she realized how different he was from other adolescent boys. He sparkled with intelligence and good humor, without the condescending posturing or corny flattery so typical of high-school athletes. He was sincerely interested in what she thought.

The teacher's arrival ended their conversation, but from then on, Manley greeted her in a more personal way.

When her romance with Jimmy Vitalla breathed its last, Jean wasn't surprised when Manley asked her out on a date. They went to a football game that weekend, then to the Blue Haven, a favorite hangout. She talked for hours with Manley, oblivious to everything around her and experiencing the delicious euphoria of young love. Their first kiss, beneath a starry autumn sky, awakened a new sense of wonder in her. Her new romance made her relationship with Jimmy seem like a mere flirtation.

Jean had two more years of high school to complete, but Manley, now nineteen years old, graduated that spring. He was called back by the army because of his excellent language skills, and he spent the next two years doing intelligence work in Germany, primarily intercepting communist radio broadcasts. Jean and Manley wrote to one another almost every day.

Shortly before Jean's graduation, Manley proposed marriage in one of his letters. He arranged for his mother to drive to Jean's house and present her with a beautiful ring to seal the engagement. Six months later, in 1952, he returned from Europe, and they were married. Jean was eighteen years old.

They set up housekeeping in a little apartment in North Adams, Massachusetts. They both worked at Sprague Electric Company—

Jean as chief clerk of the blueprint department, Manley as a technical writer.

In their fourth year of marriage, Laurie was born. Soon after, Manley enrolled in courses at Wesleyan University to pursue his ultimate goal of being a teacher. In his opinion, this was the most important job he could do.

Laurie was only seven weeks old when the Tylers moved to Durham, Connecticut, where Manley attended classes at night and worked days as a technical writer at Durham Manufacturing Company. They struggled financially but were very happy.

When Laurie was two they moved back to North Adams because Jean's mother was ill. Edith Oldham recovered, but Jean and Manley decided against moving again. Manley continued his education at North Adams State College. Employment opportunities in the area were not as plentiful as they had been in Connecticut, and Manley worked at various night and summer jobs, including pumping gas, selling cars and insurance, supervising construction, and owning a small business.

Steven was born when Laurie was seven. Jean had stopped working to raise the children, and her plans for a college degree were postponed. Manley, meanwhile, had completed a Bachelor of Arts degree in education and had begun teaching seventh grade at Clarksburg Elementary School, just north of North Adams. In that first year, Jean saw that Manley had chosen the right profession. He loved his job. It was obvious that he considered teaching to be a mission more so than an occupation. Jean was Manley's confidante for the various successes or challenges that he experienced in the classroom. He shared everything with her: the daily progress of his seventh and eighth graders and how he had won over his students and helped them to surmount obstacles. She also shared in the inevitable failures and disappointments.

After a few years of night courses, Manley earned his masters degree in education; but he never made Jean feel that her job managing the household was any less important than his own. Jean kept the family nurtured and well fed. She baked muffins every morning and pies and other sweets several times a week. Manley always went to work with a slice of fresh pie packed in his lunch. It was an idyllic existence . . . high-school sweethearts happy with each other and their life's role. They had many friends and an active social life. Their finances were stable for the first time.

Life was particularly sweet for Manley, who had experienced psychological hardship as a child. His self-involved mother never seemed to know what she wanted. When Manley was five years old, his parents divorced. His mother took Manley from Augusta, Maine, where he had been born, to her hometown of North Adams, where she left his upbringing to his grandparents. Fortunately, they were loving and generous people.

Manley's father showed even less interest in his son than his mother had. More than once he phoned from Augusta to say he was coming for a visit, and young Manley would wait for him all day on the steps of his grandparents' home. But his father never arrived.

Manley never forgot what it was like to be a vulnerable child at the mercy of events beyond his control, with disappointment at every turn. Whenever the opportunity arose to be of help to a child, he did so with all his heart.

Jean remembered one particular boy from a broken family where alcoholism and criminality were the norm. He was caught stealing money from his teacher's purse and was punished, then ostracized by teachers and students alike. It was understood that, having been branded a thief, he was never to be trusted.

Manley heard of the situation and believed it was unfair to leave the boy with no way to atone. He thus gave the boy a chance to prove he could be trusted: Manley asked the child to deliver money to the man who brought the daily newspaper to the Tyler home. The boy agreed, and every week he carried the money across town in an unsealed envelope. He never stole a penny. Thanks to Manley's compassion, the child had salvaged his self-respect.

Jean's love for Manley contained fascination. He was something of a modern-day Don Quixote, Jean thought, tilting at an ever-turning windmill of ignorance, trying to dispel some of the darkness. It was not surprising that one of his favorite songs was "The Impossible Dream" from the show *Man of La Mancha*. It held special meaning for him, as if the lyrics had sprung from his own life.

Jean was particularly proud of Manley's accomplishments because, in comparison to her own happy childhood, his was fraught with so many obstacles. Jean was the only child of Joe and Edith Oldham, and all of her aunts and uncles showered her with love as she grew up. She was used to having her slightest wish acted on by the doting adults around her. Once she mentioned that she might like to have a ski jacket, and a week later she was presented with an entire ski outfit, including boots and hat, which they had all chipped in to buy. She was used to being the center of attention. When she was small, the family would parade her in front of other adults, showing off how smart and pretty she was. Once, in her parents' living room, they stood her on top of a table, and she sang while everyone applauded.

She was never a spoiled child, however. Her parents were strict but fair. She was especially close with her father, a gentle, loving soul with the simple yet profound wisdom of a man with an unshakable sense of what was right and wrong and whose happiness stemmed from making others happy. . . .

Like her father, Jean realized now, Manley tended to view things in terms of ethical and moral stances, in black and white, particularly when the welfare of children was involved, and she could imagine his rubbing certain people—teachers, other staff members, the school board—the wrong way because of it. Whatever the cause of his current unhappiness at work, she was optimistic that it would end soon. Summer vacation would do him good. He could catch up on the reading he'd started over the winter, play the radio, and putter around in the basement making things out of wood.

Jean heard the paperboy ride by on his bike and fling their paper into their driveway. She went outside and retrieved it. As she stood up with it, she saw Steven turn the corner at the end of the street and pedal his bicycle toward home.

She went into the house and brought the newspaper to Manley. Laurie had gone upstairs.

"Steven's coming," Jean called to her husband.

By the time Manley got to the kitchen, Steven was bursting in. "Hi, Dad!"

Manley hugged and lifted the eight-year-old with a laugh as Buttons and Babe barked around them. "Hi, partner! What've you been up to?"

"Playin' ball."

Manley put the boy down, so the dogs could have their time with Steven. Manley stood still in the center of the room and waited.

"Let's have a catch, Dad," Steven suggested.

"Great."

The boy ran upstairs to get a baseball, while Manley went into his bedroom and changed into blue jeans and a sweatshirt. Then he took his baseball glove from the hallway closet and headed outside.

Steven was waiting for him. Manley raised his glove, and the boy immediately threw the hardball. It hit Manley's glove with a sharp thud, dead center, chest high. He grinned and threw it back.

Jean went outside and watched, leaning against the corner of the house. The breeze pulled at her blue cotton dress and mussed her short brown hair. Manley and Steven jogged to the open field beyond the yard.

"Throw one up high, Dad!"

Manley laughed and sent one up, a dark dot against cottony clouds. It hung for a second as Steven maneuvered under it.

"Good catch, Steven!" Manley yelled.

"Another one, Dad. Send one to the moon!"

Manley looked at the sky, reared back, and threw the ball with all his might. It shot straight up, so high that it shrank to a barely visible speck. It drifted back toward the houses.

"Wow!" Steven yelled. Keeping his eye on the speck, he ran to his right, close to a neighbor's forsythia bush, as the baseball hurtled toward him.

Apprehensive, Manley ran forward and shouted, "Watch out, Steven!"

The boy ignored the warning, stayed with the ball into the bush, and caught it.

Jean let out the breath she had been holding. She and Manley exchanged looks of relief.

"He's your son," Jean quipped, as if Steven's bravado were out of her hands.

"You had something to do with it," Manley defended.

"Yeah, but you're the coach."

"That's true," Manley agreed. He turned to Steven. "That was quite a catch, Steven. But this isn't a real game. And you're just a kid."

"I'm big enough," Steven said.

Manley looked at his wife with a smile and shrugged. Jean was glad to see him relaxed.

Laurie appeared on the side steps. "Let's play whiffle ball," she called.

"Yeah!" yelled Steven. "I'm pitching."

Laurie ran to get the plastic bat and ball, and Jean went inside to lower the heat on the simmering beef and change into shirt, jeans, and sneakers.

As always, the teams were Steven and Jean against Laurie and Manley. They played happily for almost an hour in the intoxicatingly mild springtime air. Jean and Laurie were good players, though Manley and Steven's experience in hitting showed. They all played to win, but mostly they yelled and laughed.

31

Finally Jean decided to get the meal ready. Laurie went with her to help, while Manley and Steven stayed out as long as they could, until they were called inside for dinner.

* * *

That night, in a mood of dread, Manley drove the short distance back to the school. He parked and walked through the deepening dusk toward the brick building, steeling himself for what he had to do.

The office where the school-committee members, superintendent, and principal met twice a month was charged with the expectancy of a courtroom and a heavy inevitability.

All three members of the school board had decided to approve tenure for eighth-grade teacher Bruce Walsh against Manley's protests, and now they found it embarrassing to face the principal. Art Brul—, chairman of the school committee and an old friend of the Tyler family's, felt particularly awkward. Young Walsh might be confrontational and abrasive, but neither Art nor the other board members had heard evidence that the instructor had acted unethically or incompetently.

It hurt Art to go against Manley, but under the circumstances he saw no other choice. Why, he wondered, had Manley taken such drastic measures? Hadn't he realized that there was no reason to deny tenure? Manley had always been self-controlled; he had always known exactly what he was doing. But Bruce Walsh had somehow gotten to him, causing him to lose all perspective.

Something was odd about the whole situation; it was bizarre that Manley had let personal animosity get the better of him. This was not the Manley whom Art had known since grammar school. He wondered if the rumors circulating for two weeks were true. Was Manley going to resign? *We'll find out tonight,* Art thought sadly.

The meeting lacked the usual friendly chatter. They were all on edge, remembering the previous meeting, when Walsh had challenged his principal's negative evaluation.

Manley nodded to everyone as he took his seat, but he spoke to no one. He waited stoically for everyone to get settled and watched the men he had thought of as friends. He waited patiently as they conducted regular business. He even answered questions and added his own point of view when asked.

At the appropriate time he made his brief announcement: "I regret to say that I've decided to resign as principal."

The faces in the room showed no surprise, and this acted as confirmation to Manley that he had decided correctly. He didn't trust himself to say anything more, so he rose and walked to Art Brulé, then handed him a letter from his inner pocket:

Dear Mr. Brulé:

I would like to resign from the position of principal of the Clarksburg Schools as of the beginning of the 1971 – 72 school year in September.

I have not been happy as a principal and I do not care for the type of work involved. I miss the classroom a great deal and I much prefer teaching over being a principal. If you recall, I turned in a resignation last spring but when it was torn up another year was to be tried. This time it has to be a firm decision.

I was much more successful in the classroom and that is really where my interest is. I would like to apply for one of the teaching openings that you will have in the middle to upper grades.

Sincerely yours,
Manley A. Tyler

Art's heavy sigh was unnaturally loud in the uncomfortable silence. The board members all read the strangely awkward letter in turn. There were a couple of questions put to Manley about his reasons, but he didn't want to discuss it beyond saying that he harbored no animosity and wished them well in their search for a new principal.

When the meeting was adjourned he made his way out of the room with as much dignity as his wobbly legs and the pressure in his chest would allow. He quickened his pace out of the building and to his car. Instead of going straight home, he drove around aimlessly for a long time.

The children were asleep and Jean was reading a mystery novel on the couch in the den when Manley returned home. She put the book aside and met him in the kitchen. He returned her kiss perfunctorily and went to the kitchen table. He sank down heavily, avoiding her eyes. He hadn't removed his coat.

"I resigned tonight."

"No!" She backed up, leaned against the refrigerator, and stared at him. She couldn't think because of the sudden vacuum in her stomach.

"It's true. I did it." Manley continued without emotion, "This time it's for real. My mind is made up."

Jean found her voice. "Why?"

"I just can't take it anymore."

"I don't understand. Do you want to teach again? Did you tell them you wanted to be in the classroom again?"

"It was in the letter, but they won't hire me. The superintendent told me last week that he was against my teaching in the same district. We never did get along."

"Do you have a job in mind somewhere else?"

"No."

"Why not? You could name your spot. I'm sure any school system would be glad to have you."

"I'll get another job. I have plenty of time. I'll finish up the year." To avoid further questions, he got up and hung his coat in the hall closet.

Jean felt sick in her stomach. She shivered. She sat at the table, feeling suddenly old. *He knows what he's doing. He must have his reasons.* But she couldn't imagine what they might be. Why would he give up the career he loved?

Manley had disappeared into their bedroom at the end of the hall. She followed and found him sitting on the edge of the bed, casually taking off his tie.

"Are you going to tell me what's going on?" she demanded.

He looked straight ahead, and the movements of his hands stopped. In a composed voice he said, "I've been giving this a lot of thought. The pressure has been building up, and I realized I had to do it. It's time I made a career change, that's all."

Jean shook her head, trying to excise the weird unreality that was fogging her mind. "This isn't like you, Manley. Why let one incident disrupt your whole career?"

"I just don't want to be principal anymore."

"Manley," Jean implored desperately, "please help me to understand. Has something happened that you haven't told me about?" Her voice had risen in pitch and volume.

For the first time he looked at her, furious. "I've told you everything. Why would I *hide* anything from you?"

Jean was stunned by his sudden anger. She felt as if he'd struck her in the face. They had been married nineteen years, and she couldn't remember the last time he had turned on her. But his face was stiff, his eyes dark and determined. She had no choice but to drop the subject.

"I'm sorry," she said. "It's just that I didn't see this coming."
He looked away without speaking.

She got up. She had to move, do something, anything. "You didn't eat your dessert before. Want some now? It's cherry pie."

"I guess so." He followed her into the kitchen.

She brought him a wedge of pie and poured him a glass of milk. He took a bite, and she felt better just watching him eat. But her mind continued to search for some explanation to cling to. Maybe he was undergoing some fundamental change; she knew people sometimes reacted strangely as middle age approached. Perhaps his dissatisfaction with being a principal had prompted him to consider other careers. He had always thrived on challenge; he might yearn for something different. But he had always carefully planned his moves and thought things out in meticulous detail before taking action. And he had always discussed his ideas with her. This secretiveness, like his anger, was entirely new.

They went to bed soon after. She reached for him, wondering if he would pull away, still smoldering with that strange anger; but he didn't. He turned to her and kissed her on the forehead and drew her to him in a tight embrace.

Jean's whisper was almost a whimper. "I don't know what to think of all this, Manley."

"I know." He sounded like his old reassuring self, and she felt better. She waited for him to explain, now that they lay in the warm safety of their own bed. For a long while he said nothing.

Finally she asked, "What am I going to tell the kids?"

After a long pause he said, "Just assure them that everything will be all right."

"But it's so unlike you, Manley."

"Please trust me, Jean. I won't let anything happen to us. Sometimes these things happen. Just don't worry."

In the morning Jean tried to be as cheerful as she could despite a fitful night's sleep that included a panic-filled nightmare.

Manley was his usual self, as if yesterday's bombshell were perfectly natural. She read in his mood an unmistakable feeling of relief. It made her wonder how long he'd been planning to resign. It bothered her deeply that he had been thinking about it for weeks, perhaps, and had not mentioned it to her.

She needed to understand. Now that they'd slept on it, she broached the subject again while he was finishing breakfast.

"You've been planning this for some time, haven't you, dear? You could have told me. You know I want only what's best for you."

"Of course I know that. I just didn't want to be talked out of it again, like last year." He bit into a muffin.

"So you have an idea what you're going to do next?"

He didn't meet her gaze, but stared down into the table as he chewed slowly. "Don't worry. Have I ever had trouble finding work? I'll probably have a hard time deciding which offer to accept when they start coming in."

"Yes, but you can understand *my* concern, can't you?"

"Sure."

Why is this so difficult? she wondered. "Do you want to go back to teaching?"

"That's a possibility. We'll see."

She waited patiently for him to continue, but he concentrated on chewing his last slice of bacon.

She tried once more. "If it's a matter of moving away, Manley, the kids and I could handle that. It would be difficult for them, but they're solid kids—they'll adapt. I don't want you to have to do something you're not happy with."

He rose from the table. "I'll be late." Seeing her frustrated expression, he added, "It'll be fine. You'll see." He put on his blazer.

His false calm infuriated her. This was her family, too. She had to know what to do, what to plan for. "Can't you see that it's confusing for me? All of a sudden you have these deep, dark secrets—"

He was moving toward the door with his briefcase. When he whirled to face her, the cold fury in his eyes chilled her to speechlessness.

"What more do you want from me?" he hissed. "I can't explain everything that happens. I can't know what other people are thinking. It's useless to go on and on complaining. I want to forget about it. I just want to forget about it. Is that too much to ask?"

She stared at him, trying to contain her fright. Wordlessly she watched him walk outside while her stomach reacted to the fear that engulfed her.

Manley got into his car and drove away, but Jean continued standing by the door. No matter how she looked at it, she couldn't grasp why Manley, with his tenacious sense of purpose, would quit a job he'd worked so hard to attain, regardless of who was making it hard for him. He had a will of steel and was so bright that obstacles didn't long thwart him. His behavior was so uncharacteristic that it struck her as an elaborate prank. Soon someone would lower the curtain and turn on the lights.

She was sitting at the kitchen table staring at nothing when her daughter came downstairs a few minutes later.

"What's going on, Mom?" Laurie whispered nervously. "Why was Dad angry with you?"

Jean didn't want to worry her daughter unnecessarily, but she had to be truthful. "Your father resigned as principal yesterday."

"What?" Laurie's eyes came fully awake with surprise. "Why?" Her voice was rising in pitch, much as Jean's had the night before. "He's a great principal. Everyone loves him."

"Apparently some people have been giving him trouble, and he . . . can't or won't put up with it anymore." She tried a smile, but Laurie wasn't fooled.

"What's going to happen, Mom?"

Jean shook her head resignedly. "I guess he'll get another job."

"As a principal somewhere else?"

"I don't know." Jean willed herself out of her shock. "Is Steven up yet?"

"I think so."

"Have something to eat. Those muffins are still warm. It's getting late." She looked fondly at Laurie as she got up to make sure Steven was getting ready for school. "Don't worry, sweetheart. It'll work out. You'll see."

The news of Manley Tyler's resignation was in the North Adams *Transcript* the following Monday and an article in the larger Pittsfield, Massachusetts, *Berkshire Eagle* as well. Manley's acquaintances were quoted as saying how sorry they were to see him go and how good he'd been for the school system. There was puzzled speculation on why he was leaving. A reporter phoned and wanted to talk to Manley, but he declined, stating that his reasons were personal.

Jean was not surprised by the stir his unexpected resignation had created in the community. It made her feel good that people still supported and admired him. His record as an educator was something to be proud of, and people wouldn't soon forget it.

May passed uneventfully into June. Jean's world had wobbled monumentally on its axis and left the family changed, but the summer stretched invitingly before them. She looked forward to the healing peace of togetherness. She tamed her fears into submission and was committed to shielding the children from uncertainty as much as possible. Steven, being so young, was barely aware of the change.

Jean nurtured the hope that this period was merely an abrupt transition, one of life's occasional surprises that seemed worse than it actually was.

After the first shock, life resumed normally enough for Jean to wonder if she had overreacted. Manley was relaxed and confident. He'd already begun his search for another job with a typical display of methodical organization. As a result, Jean, too, relaxed, pushing any residual misgivings into the deepest chambers of her mind.

Laurie was old enough to feel afraid. She knew how hard her parents had toiled and sacrificed to get where they were. As a young child she had watched her father working and going to school, staying up nights to write papers and to study for exams. She knew that as a child, she had been fed expensive cuts of beef while her parents had made do with chicken. She had shared their triumph when her father attained his goals and went beyond them until, three years before, their finances allowed the family to build the modest home where they now lived. How could her father toss it away on a whim?

Although Laurie saw her mother minimizing the effects, she perceived the true depth of Jean's terror. Laurie took cues from her mother and acted as if everything was normal, but inside she felt adrift and vulnerable. Habitually she said prayers each morning and before she went to sleep at night. Now she prayed fervently that her father would get another job. She cried herself to sleep every night worrying about it.

On his very last day at Clarksburg Elementary School, Principal Manley Tyler wandered the empty halls and rooms, light-headed from emotions so conflicted he couldn't control them. The students had departed days before, and he had spent the intervening time wrapping things up for his successor. He was hopeful that he was leaving his problems behind him.

His footsteps echoed through halls still hung with the primitive artwork of students. A seeming lifetime of memories inhabited the corridors, perceivable in quiet moments like this, when the educational engine of the school was idle. He knew the rooms of this building as well as the rooms of his own home. He had shared time with so many young lives; he had loved so many children. And they'd loved him. So many that their names blurred in his mind— but their spirits glowed with identity.

The pain of separation was fierce. It had been a decade filled with singing, shouting, laughing, and countless expressions of revelation on beautiful young faces as understanding of new concepts dawned.

He wandered and cried, hearing his own sobs down the halls. This was what it had all come to: this moment in an empty school, weeping like a hurt, confused child looking for his mother. This was the culmination of his long-fought, illustrious career.

Why?

After a while he wound up in the gym. He looked around for a basketball, but the room was bare. He turned and went out through the doors and broke into a run. His basketball, the only thing he hadn't packed, was in his office closet.

He returned to the gym. His first shot went in, then his second. He dribbled away and spun as he jumped, letting the ball fly. It went in . . . then another and another, shot with feeling, with defiance, as he focused his mind on the net.

An hour later Bill, the custodian, looked in, wondering who was in the gym. When he saw Manley, he waved. "Hello, Mr. Tyler!"

The principal waved back, but the custodian couldn't read the look on his face. He backed out of the gym and left Manley alone. He seemed to want it that way.

As he walked back toward the front of the school Bill continued to hear the basketball's rhythmic thumping on the gym floor, then a pause for a shot, then more thumping.

CHAPTER 3

Summer
1971

*O*n July Manley took Steven fishing and camping in Vermont, which allowed Jean and Laurie time to talk privately. They spoke in hushed tones over breakfast, although there was no need to be quiet.

They had been on unsure footing since Manley's resignation. Neither mother nor daughter wanted to say too much and confirm the confusion they had been feeling these last months. Yet they had a powerful need to confide in each other. Laurie was mature; even when Laurie was a child, Jean had joked that her daughter was eight going on thirty-eight.

"Please tell me what's going on, Mom. The whole thing gives me the creeps."

Jean reached across the kitchen table and put her hand over Laurie's. "We've had hard times before, dear. We can weather it."

"Then tell me."

"I'm not hiding anything from you."

"But you make it sound better than it is."

Jean smiled weakly. "I guess I tend to do that, but I'm not doing it now—honest. The sad fact is that your father hasn't told me anything more than what you already know. I really don't know what he's thinking."

Jean paused, wondering how much of her inner turmoil she should share. The hurt on Laurie's face was plain, so Jean decided to be frank.

"I keep wondering if something worse happened at the school than your dad has told us," she said. "But I haven't heard anything further about it, and I know we would have heard something if your dad was keeping something from us. I've even wondered if

40

he's having a psychological problem. His mother had a history of emotional difficulties."

"I didn't know that."

"Your father and I didn't talk about it much. She was an unstable person, under the care of doctors most of her life and medicated for nerves."

Laurie thought that over, then asked, "Is it a nervous breakdown?"

"The thought has crossed my mind, but your dad hasn't really seemed that different. He says not to worry, that everything's fine."

The expression on Laurie's face darkened. "I feel like everything's falling apart, Mom. What's going to happen?"

"I don't know, dear. But let's not jump to conclusions; there's a logical explanation for everything. We'll have to be patient and give your father time to figure things out at his own pace. Maybe when he's working again he'll feel better and get back to normal."

"I pray everyday that he'll get a job."

"He'll find something soon. You don't have to worry."

The ring of the phone broke the moment apart. Laurie answered it.

"Hi, Keith. Yes, I'm up." At the sound of her boyfriend's voice, Laurie perked up. "I'll call you right back. Bye." She hung up the phone and left the room.

Jean heard her hurrying up the stairs. A minute later Laurie was talking to Keith on her own phone.

Jean rose, poured another cup of coffee, and brought it back to the table. She was glad when she heard a laugh from upstairs and tried to lighten her own mood. After all, the summer was progressing normally enough. Manley had been busy looking for a job, sending out resumés, and going on interviews. He had a couple of strong possibilities pending with construction companies. He had been following his usual summer routine, attending Steven's Little League games and practicing the boy's pitching skills with him at home. Manley had also continued coaching baseball for the church league and played softball in the Old Timers' League, pitching, as he had for years.

Jean's only cause for concern had come at the end of June, when Manley went to see Dr. Bill Everett in Williamstown, Massachusetts, because his right arm and leg had been "feeling hot." But the physical checkup did not reveal any problems, and when the strange heat sensation had gone away a week later, Jean felt somewhat reassured.

Within an hour Laurie was dangling her legs in the warm water of the YMCA day-camp swimming pool in North Adams, where she and her boyfriend had summer jobs as counselors. Laurie had told Keith about what was going on in her family, but he didn't think the situation was as bad as Laurie imagined.

"People change jobs all the time," he had told her. "Sometimes things like that happen in all households."

Keith was like one of the Tyler family. He ate dinner with them, played whiffle ball and softball, or board games and bumper pool in the basement family room. He'd spent many hours watching sports on television while chatting with Manley, Jean, and Steven.

Laurie loved Keith. They had been going steady for a year, and she was able to pour out her thoughts while he listened patiently. But that didn't change the situation.

Now, in the company of boisterous young campers splashing in the pool, Laurie managed to push her worries to the back of her mind; but alone in bed at night, her tumultuous emotions threatened to overwhelm her. These past weeks had been unreal. Her brain stubbornly refused to accept that her father wasn't the principal anymore.

Worse, her mom seemed changed in subtle ways. She was trying to be the same, but she had lost her lightheartedness. Laurie saw that her parents weren't pulling together.

Like Keith, her girlfriends didn't understand why she took it so seriously. They said such changes were natural. She couldn't make them understand that the situation wasn't natural for *her* family.

Although her father had always been authoritative and accomplished, in the privacy of his home he openly expressed his feelings, demonstrated love without reservation, and paid close attention to his wife and children. Laurie had often seen him cry when something moved him. When President Kennedy was murdered, her father had had tears in his eyes for days.

There were an innocence and vulnerability in Manley Tyler, perceived only by her mother and her, that needed protecting. He was more kind, sensitive, and gentle than most other adults she had known. He would fight for what was right, but he never acted tough for effect.

He loved animals as much as people, and more than once Laurie had seen him pick up a spider, take it outside, and set it loose.

"Why kill it if you can save it to live another day?" he would ask. "Who's to say that its life is any less important than ours?"

42

Before her teen years, she and her father had been inseparable, just as Steven and he were now. Besides hiking, camping, and fishing, he'd take her wherever he went around town, even to semiprofessional boxing matches at the North Adams armory on Friday nights. When she was little, Manley sometimes took her with him to work. She would sit in his classroom, feeling very grown-up, with all the older kids. In later years she'd had him as a teacher, which she minded not at all. Occasionally her classmates had muttered jealously about her being his daughter, but she didn't care—he certainly didn't treat her any better than the other students; in fact she had to toe the line more, in fairness to the others.

Dad had always been synonymous with fun. He made a game of everything. At the slightest excuse he could reach into himself and summon the child who, like Peter Pan, had never completely grown up. It was a trait that made him irresistible to adults and children alike.

Dad belonged in a school with kids. To Laurie, that was an indisputable fact. She couldn't imagine him being anywhere else. Would the world ever be the same again?

Steven Tyler stared into the clear, swirling water at his feet. Beneath the surface were trout; it was a magic trick of nature's. No one had put the fish there, as they had in the bigger streams and rivers down near where everyone lived. Here, near the top of the Green Mountains, the trout just grew on their own, mysteriously, from out of the rocks and sunlight and forest debris.

He wanted to drop in his fishing line, rest, and see what would happen. He was tired from two hours of hiking, but he wouldn't complain. Eager to please, he would do exactly as his father instructed.

They had left their camp far down the mountain, where they'd stayed overnight, and would return to it at the end of the day. All they had with them now were fishing gear and a few cooking utensils. They trudged around thickets and boulders, skirting the denser undergrowth, crisscrossing the stream, climbing even higher.

The boy wondered what his dad was thinking; Manley Tyler, lost in thought, had hardly talked this morning. Steven had trouble keeping up with his father's adult pace and wished they could take it easy and just meander around, the way Steven did when he was alone in the woods. If he had complained, he knew his father would stop and rest; but Steven would have to be ready to drop to do that because the pride he saw in his father's eyes was worth

43

pushing his body till it hurt. Steven wanted to prove he was the best son his father could ever want.

There was something heart filling about the way his father stood so erect and tall, with a strong, sympathetic smile. They were buddies, and they had fun, just like when he was with his friends, only better. His buddies had often said he was lucky to have such a dad.

They reached a flat marshy area surrounded by big oaks and thin birches. At the near end of the marsh were two small pools.

Manley stopped, and Steven came up beside him. "Is this it, Dad?"

"Yes. There're just marshy springs here."

"It's neat. I bet no one ever comes here." Manley didn't answer, but Steven noticed a flicker of annoyance crossing his face. "Remember the time we surprised those two deer, Dad?" He looked up at his father, who was not listening. "One made that squawk sound, remember? You'd never heard a deer make that sound before. Remember?"

Manley looked bored. "Yes, I remember. Now could you be quiet? Any deer are gone by now with all your yapping."

Steven felt his throat constrict. His father had never spoken to him like that before. He stared in wide-eyed confusion, trying to understand what was wrong. "I'm sorry, Dad."

Without saying anything his father walked away, sat down on a log, and began checking his fishing gear. Steven stood still for a few moments, then sat down quietly beside him.

They sat for a while, then Manley took a sandwich from his pocket and bit into it. Then he seemed to remember his son and offered him the other half. Steven chewed slowly, imitating his father.

Dad must not feel well, he thought. "Do you have a headache?" he asked carefully.

"No." Manley stared straight ahead and chewed.

After a few minutes his father's mood changed, and they began enjoying themselves. To Steven, it was as if the sun had come out again. They continued hiking, casting in here and there. The bushes thinned, and Steven and Manley came out on a shelf of rock three feet above a large pool. Steven could see nothing below the surface of the water because of the mottled reflection of sunlight through the trees. They baited their hooks and cast out. Nothing happened at first as they experimented with casting and working their worms across the pool in different patterns. When Steven brought his hook out to check it, Manley offered his own pole for his son to try. Steven accepted gladly. As he dragged the line toward him, he felt a sharp tug. He reeled in, and a large rainbow trout broke the surface with splash and spray.

"I got one!" the boy shrieked, and yanked it toward himself, almost hitting his father with the fish. It was a nine-inch beauty, with a stripe along its side and multicolored spots.

"Good fish, Steven! We'll definitely keep it. Careful you don't drop it—it won't bite again if it falls back in."

Manley held the pole while Steven took the hook out of the trout's mouth. It struggled valiantly, and he barely got it into the creel as it slipped from his small hands.

Manley laughed and mussed his son's hair. "He's a strong one . . . so beautiful it's a shame to see him die."

"Should we throw him back?" Steven didn't want to; this was a trophy worth keeping.

"It's up to you, Steven. He's yours."

Steven looked into his father's eyes for a moment, then reached for the fish and tossed it back into the pool. It vanished in a flash of silver.

Manley rested his hand on his son's shoulder. The glow of approval in his eyes bestowed honor on him. Steven's radiant smile beamed from a dirty face scratched by branches. "You're a great kid, Steven. The best."

"So're you, Dad."

Manley sighed deeply. "What a team."

Steven was glad he had thrown back the fish because his father was back to his old self. They caught a few more in the next hour— or his father did. Steven got a couple of throw backs, but when Manley let him use his pole again, Steven was surprised to catch another good fish right away. That had happened quite a few times in the past, too. Then it dawned on Steven that his father knew he had a fish on the line before he handed over the pole.

Manley sent Steven to gather dry sticks for a fire while he cleaned the fish carefully. Soon the trout was sputtering in the pan.

Steven couldn't imagine anything better than this. He slipped into reverie, in which he and his father were pioneer woodsmen alone in the wild, living off the land, watchful of predatory animals and thieves. Indians were friendly because his father was famous among them as a teacher-protector who respected their ways and learned from them. Side by side they bravely faced dangers but lived in harmony with the wild animals of the forest. They could take care of themselves.

Laurie had returned home and was sitting with Jean on lawn chairs behind the house when Steven and Manley got home. They got up and came over to the car.

"Hi, Hon." Jean kissed her husband.

"Catch any fish?" asked Laurie.

"Sure," Steven said. "What do you think? We ate most of them, but we still have a couple."

Manley gave his daughter a hug. "Hi, Laur. Missed you. How come you never come fishing anymore? We had fun."

She laughed. "I have a job—can't go traipsing off into the woods whenever I feel like it."

"I suppose not." He kissed her on the head, then turned to Jean. "Did anyone call while we were away?"

"No."

Manley opened the trunk of the car and took out the tent and sleeping bags. After setting them on the ground, he looked around the backyard. "Where's that son of ours? He jumps ship as soon as we pull in."

"He was thirsty," Jean answered. "He went straight for the lemonade. The next stop was the bathroom."

Manley laughed.

At the sound of the phone ringing, Manley sprinted into the house. Jean could hear his voice through the open window.

"Hello. This *is* Manley Tyler. Yes." A pause. "Yes, how are you Mr. Moore?" A long silence, then, "Excellent. I'd be happy to. Yes. Not at all, no. Next week. Very good. I'll be there. Yes. Thanks again, Mr. Moore. Good-bye."

"Who was it?" Jean asked as he came back out.

"I've got a job." His broad smile was jubilant.

Laurie popped out of her chair. "Where, Dad?"

"Not far from here. Bear Swamp. They're building a hydroelectric plant. A big project."

"Yippee!" Laurie let out her relief in that one sound.

Jean laughed happily, and Steven came out of the house. "Dad's got a job," she told him.

"Are you gonna be a teacher again, Dad?"

"No. Daddy's going to work on a hydroelectric plant," Laurie said impatiently.

"A what?"

"Big machines that generate electricity, using running water, like a river," Manley explained.

"How do you know about that stuff, Dad?"

"Well, this is a little new to me, but it's basically construction, and I worked in construction before you were born."

"Yeah? With cranes and bulldozers and everything?"

"Sure." Manley laughed. He looked more relaxed than Jean had seen him look in months.

They all asked more questions about the new job, and he told them what he knew. Then he said, "How about celebrating? Let's take a ride down to McDonald's."

"Yay!" Laurie and Steven both shouted their approval.

Jean loved their trips to McDonald's—it was one of Manley's favorite things to do, and besides, it meant that she could stow the fish in the freezer. She might even get away with giving them to a neighbor.

The twenty-five mile ride to Pittsfield, Massachusetts, was a family show-on-wheels. Led by Manley's booming baritone and punctuated by Steven's silly shenanigans, they sang songs in a riotous party mood the whole way.

Jean allowed herself to feel optimistic. Whatever had gone wrong at the school was over now. This was the beginning of a new chapter. She would put aside the question of why Manley was leaving education; he would tell her all about it when he was ready—he always did. One of the songs Manley boomed was an old favorite that she hadn't heard him sing in a long time:

> *"C'mon along and let the wedding chimes,*
> *Bring happy times/For Mandy and me!"*

The following week Manley started his new job as assistant supervisor of the engineering staff at the Bear Swamp construction project. Jean could tell he felt good about the position; it even paid more money than he'd earned as a school principal.

During their marriage Manley and Jean had had a habit of sitting together in the kitchen and talking after the children were in bed. It was a time when their friendship could express itself freely, and they could air their thoughts in privacy. Since his resignation from Clarksburg, Jean had missed something in her relationship with her husband, which she felt most poignantly in these moments alone together. He hadn't been confiding his innermost feelings to her, and she missed the commitment to honesty that had been the cornerstone of their relationship from the beginning. She had been patient, allowing him time to sort things out for himself during this transition. Now that he had started a new career, she expected him to open up.

One night over milk and cookies she asked him about his new job.

"It's fine. A nice bunch of guys," he said.

"How does it feel being back in a construction job after all these years?"

"Not bad."

"But how do you *feel?* Do you miss being with children?"

"A little."

He was complacent and closemouthed, and Jean wondered why. "That's *it?* You have no other feelings about things?"

"What else do you want?"

"You used to tell me all about your jobs, Manley. You've told me almost nothing about this one. Do you like your boss?"

"Sure. We get along fine."

He still doesn't get it, she thought, dismayed.

"Manley, why is it we never seem to talk anymore?"

"Of course we talk."

"No . . . I mean you don't tell me things the way you used to. You really used to talk about your work, not just say things like 'It's fine.' Why aren't you sharing your feelings with me?"

He looked at her with expressionless eyes. "I don't know what you mean."

She sighed heavily and plunged in. "You know, you never told me why you resigned. I've been waiting for you to tell me. What happened that hurt you so much?" She waited, but he stared into the tabletop.

At last he said, "I just couldn't put up with all the baloney anymore."

"Gossip and infighting? That never bothered you before. There must have been more to it. I know you, Manley. I can tell that something deeper was involved."

In the stillness she could hear his breathing and the hum of the electric clock. He took a deep breath, got up abruptly, went to the window, and looked out into the dark. Without turning he spoke emotionlessly. "I wanted a total change."

This was not her husband of twenty years. Frustration made her desperate. She said to his back: "What good am I if you can't tell me everything?"

He roused himself and turned toward her. His eyes were hard and flat. "I think you're overreacting."

"But don't you remember the way we used to be, Manley? Please don't close me out. I can't take it!"

But there was a wall around him that might as well have been made of granite.

She closed her eyes sadly. "What happened? What turned you against me?"

He shook his head in emphatic negation. "Against you? Never." He watched her, then sought the blackness beyond the window again. He seemed to absorb some of its gloom. Barely stifling his animosity, he said into the glass, "Why are you *picking* at me? Picking, picking, all the time! With all the problems I've had, the last thing I need is one more!"

Jean hung her head, giving in to a fatigue and loneliness that emptied her of any remaining energy. She could only manage a weak, "Sorry."

She sat there, afraid to say anything, unable to think, feeling helpless against a malevolent confusion that threatened the sanctuary of her life.

CHAPTER 4

Summer 1972 – Winter 1973

Overseeing the welfare of her family had been delightfully easy for Jean in the past. As the months passed, it had grown more complicated. The rock-solid framework that their lives had been built upon had eroded. She had no choice but to continue living day-to-day, dealing as best she could. She kept the peace with Manley at all costs and was patient with him. He refused to reveal his feelings, and she did not press him. She didn't want to drive him even farther from her.

What a difference from the way he used to be, she often thought. Every time she stopped to think about how their marriage had changed, she was forced to fight her despair.

Jean still believed that before long Manley would be back to his old self. Her misgivings about his behavior did not weaken her support of him. If his behavior had a psychological basis, there was no telling what could happen; but he was a truly good man, and if he was going through a difficult time, she was absolutely certain that it was through no fault of his own. Come what may, she would not let anything destroy the love that had existed between them since their adolescence.

Jean had not held a job since Laurie was born, but the uncertainties of the immediate future turned her thoughts to practical matters of survival. After Manley was settled into his new job, Jean studied newspaper want ads. She applied at the First Agricultural Bank, took an exam, and was pleasantly surprised to be offered a job as teller.

By mid-August Jean was a working woman, but the job was not to last long. In the fall of 1972 her father, Joe Oldham, underwent a hernia operation and abnormalities were found. After further tests it was determined that he had a malignancy.

50

Jean's mother, Edith, had been slowly recuperating from the removal of a tumor in her leg, and since Edith was still not well, Jean quit her job and went with her father to Boston, where the closest facility equipped for administering radiation treatment was located.

Joe Oldham died of leukemia in July 1973.

The family gathered at Edith's home after the funeral. Jean, knowing that Manley would have to take a few days off from work, took him aside.

"Dear, you'd better call Bear Swamp and let them know."

"Oh? Yes. I'll call." He disappeared into the kitchen. Jean went back into the living room where everyone was talking quietly. After a while, when Manley didn't appear, she looked in on him. He was in an agitated state, and the contents of his wallet were strewn over the kitchen table.

"What are you looking for?" she asked.

He looked up nervously. "I can't find it."

"What?"

"The phone number where I work."

"Maybe we can get the number from information."

Manley had a puzzled look. "I can't think of the name of my boss." He got red in the face.

"Oh, come on, Manley. Surely you know the name of your boss."

"I don't," he said. "It's completely slipped my mind."

She shook her head with annoyance. She didn't have time for this now. "What's his first name?"

His expression was blank.

She waited.

He started looking through the folded papers on the table, then searched through the wallet again, but came up empty. Then he began going through his pockets.

Jean watched him, disbelieving. Everyone had loved her father, Manley not the least of them. *Poor man,* she thought. *He's more distracted than I am.* "Manley, forget it for now. We'll get the number later." She began helping him to gather his papers.

When they were back at home, Manley still couldn't come up with his boss's name. Jean remembered that an old friend's cousin worked at the Bear Swamp project, too. "I'll call Angie Potter and get Eddie's number. He works on the same job, right?"

"Yes."

Angie gave Jean her cousin's number, and Manley finally notified his boss that he'd be taking time off for the death in the family.

Jean attributed Manley's momentary difficulty to the emotional upheaval. Her own grief clouded the situation for some time. With her father gone and Manley not quite himself, Jean felt deprived of her two most solid supporters.

Once again she looked for work. She found a job at Lamb Printing Company, a small family-owned printer in North Adams. The patriarch, Victor Lamb,Sr., had just retired, but his son Bill managed the concern with flexibility and understanding. Jean had intended to work part-time, but within weeks she was working full-time and enjoying the camaraderie and family atmosphere at the old business.

A New England snowstorm raged outside, buffeting the house. Ten-year-old Steven Tyler had walked through the stinging snow from the school-bus drop-off, and a puddle formed where he'd left his wet boots to dry by the side door. Now he sat in the kitchen of his empty home, drinking milk and eating a piece of homemade pie as he waited for his father to arrive from work.

When he heard a car drive up and shut off, he ran to the door to greet his father.

"Hi, Dad. Isn't it great outside?"

"It's blowing something awful." Manley came in and shut the door. Out of habit Steven expected a hug but was not surprised when his father's body language rebuffed him—he was getting used to it.

"Where's Laurie?" Manley asked without looking at his son.

"At Keith's. She's going to do her homework there."

Manley leaned against the wall, took off his boots, and placed them beside Steven's. Then he removed his coat and went to the hall closet with it.

"Isn't it great?" Steven asked, looking out the window. "We're supposed to get ten inches." Now that his father was home, the house felt cozy again.

Returning to the kitchen, his father answered, "It's not great for those of us who have to work."

Steven looked up, suddenly fearful. What had he said wrong? He couldn't get used to his father's mood swings when they were alone together. His mother didn't get home till an hour and a half after his father, and in the hours he and his father spent with each other every afternoon, Steven had often experienced disturbing disorientation. He and his father were no longer buddies. His father seemed old and crotchety. The boy quietly took his glass and dish to the sink.

"Want some pie, Dad?" he asked. "There's some in the refrigerator." He looked furtively at his father, his hand on the refrigerator door.

Manley didn't answer. He had lowered himself into a chair at the table and was staring out at the storm. To Steven, his father's face looked strange, with an empty expression that made him look like someone else.

"Want some? Huh, Dad?"

"What?" Manley asked, still looking at the storm.

"Want some pumpkin pie? It's good."

His father reluctantly turned toward him and sighed. "Okay." He went to the stove and made coffee while Steven put the remainder of the pie on the table. Then he got a small plate, a knife, and a fork and placed them on the table near the dish. He looked around to see if there was anything else he could do for his dad. But something about the way his father was ignoring him prompted Steven to leave the room. He turned on the television in the den.

"Damn!" Manley cried out from the kitchen.

Steven came running. His father was in the middle of the room. Anger contorted his face. "Why can't you take your boots off when you get in? Look at the puddle you left! Right in the middle of the room!" Manley hopped over to the table, threw himself into one of the chairs, and snatched impatiently at his wet sock.

"I'm sorry, Dad."

"Sorry? Don't be sorry. Do things right to begin with. Other people have to live in this house besides you."

The boy quickly got some paper towels, sank to his knees, and mopped up the water, making certain he got every drop. Without looking at his father, he threw the wet paper away in the garbage can under the sink. He wanted to bolt from the room but didn't dare until he knew Manley was satisfied. He waited and glanced at his father, who was muttering and watching him with lingering irritation.

"Did you get it all?" Manley asked.

"Yes." Steven's throat clenched and burned, an all-too-familiar feeling recently. He waited for a moment, feeling the beginning of tears.

Manley didn't notice; he left the room and made his way into the master bedroom.

Steven walked back into the den and turned off the television. Before his father could return, he went upstairs to his room and turned on his own small television.

From his bed he stared at the screen's images, but his mind remained downstairs with his father. His best friend, the one he had the most *fun* with, used to be his dad. Now Steven felt frightened of him and couldn't understand why. And his father was mean only when they were alone together.

When Steven had asked his mother why Dad was cruel to him sometimes, she had looked at him as if she thought he was making it up. She and his sister acted as if he was to blame. He thought about his behavior: He got on his father's nerves without knowing why. Sometimes it was something he did, sometimes something he didn't do; or maybe it was something he said or didn't say.

So, not understanding the new rules at all, the boy tried all the harder to please his father and waited for him to return to his old self.

CHAPTER 5

1974

*B*y the end of 1973 the construction of the Bear Swamp hydroelectric plant was nearing completion. Manley's firm had no other work in western Massachusetts at the time, but they offered some of their employees, including Manley, an opportunity to transfer to a major new project in West Germany.

Relocating was a hot topic of discussion in the Tyler household for weeks. Everyone except Manley was enthusiastic. The opportunity seemed like a ray of hope, a new adventure to experience as a family. Manley's being so cautious puzzled Jean. He had spent years in southern Germany with army intelligence and had loved it. He often spoke nostalgically of his experiences there.

It sounded like a great adventure to Laurie and Steven, even though they'd miss their friends.

Although Manley said he was weighing the pros and cons, Jean could see that he did not want to go. She knew he wouldn't get any other job offers that good, so she urged him to accept. He would earn a higher salary than he'd ever made before, with many fringe benefits. All travel and moving expenses would be paid by the construction company.

"How about the kids?" Manley reminded. "It'll take them away from friends and relatives."

"Is this my Manley I'm hearing?" Jean responded kiddingly. "The same man who used to say that children benefit from travel, that experiencing other cultures expands their horizons?"

"Steven's only a child," he said without humor.

"He wants to go. Steven can make friends anywhere. So can Laurie. This is a great opportunity."

"I'll get work with another company," he answered stubbornly.

"Of course you will," she said soothingly. "I'm surprised that you don't want to go, though. I thought you loved Germany."

"I do. I do. But we just built the house."

"With what they'll be paying you, we could buy another when we get back and have a nice nest egg tucked away. Don't forget we'll have two kids to send to college."

He didn't say anything for a long moment.

"Well?" she asked.

"I'll think it over."

Jean went with him to the final meeting with a company representative, whose words encouraged her. But watching her husband's reactions to what was said, Jean had a sinking feeling. It was clear that they wouldn't be going.

Manley confirmed his decision later in the day, but without any clear-cut reasons. He just didn't want to go, and that was that.

Jean Tyler's happy past drifted ever farther behind her. Happiness seemed curiously distant, remembered but not renewed. She was adapting to change, to a husband who never quite returned to the man he had been.

Meanwhile she carried on, her worries increasingly focused on finances. Manley's job at Bear Swamp ended in February 1974. In March he found work with a construction contractor building a new high school in North Adams. His position did not have the same degree of responsibility as he'd enjoyed at Bear Swamp, and the pay was a lot less. Jean was glad she had a steady job of her own. The family needed her income, and more than once she thought bitterly: *We spent all those years scrimping and saving and paying off his education so he could teach, and now all that seems like wasted energy.*

Manley complained about the shoddy building practices of his new employer; it irked him all the more since the building was to house children. Soon he was demoted to helping with surveying. Again his pay went down.

Jean assumed his demotion had to do with his criticisms of the company. Manley could be discreet, but when he considered something important, such as the welfare of children, he could be boldly outspoken.

Jean suffered real shock when Manley suddenly quit his job in July, after only four months. She demanded an explanation, but he was closemouthed about it. Jean didn't know what to make of it.

From what she gathered, he might have been fired or forced to resign.

Manley knew how important his income was, she thought. How could he have acted so irresponsibly? Jean was at a total loss. A recurring thought was that he might be under more mental stress than the family realized. Was he heading for a nervous breakdown? Again she remembered his mother's emotional instability. After she had divorced her husband and left young Manley to be raised by his grandparents, she drifted from relationship to relationship, with no direction in her life. She had had a prescription-drug dependency for many years before her death.

Manley, mentally unstable? Three years before she would have laughed at the idea.

Manley collected unemployment insurance and looked for work elsewhere. After a month he found a job with another construction company, which was erecting a new high-rise dormitory for North Adams State College. His earnings continued at the same mediocre level, for her college-educated husband was only a rodman with a surveying team.

"What does a rodman do?" Laurie asked her mother.

"Not much," Jean answered. "According to your uncle Bob, a rodman stands with a rod while the other surveyors take sightings."

"That's *all* Dad does? Hold a rod?"

"Apparently. It's no wonder he's earning so little money."

Jean and Laurie both worked at being as stoic and optimistic as possible. But they had the increasing need to unburden themselves to each other. When Manley rejected the opportunity to work in Germany, it had triggered a downturn in the morale of the family. The poor jobs he'd had since that time had made his decision appear even worse.

The look in Laurie's eyes was as haunted as her mother's. "He must be able to get *something* better than that. Isn't he worried about money?"

"Yes, he's worried more now than ever. That's why it's so peculiar that he can't seem to get a better job. If there are none available, then we'll move. We can't go on like *this* for the rest of our lives."

"He doesn't want to move."

"I know. I hate to say this—and don't you mention it to him— but I think he needs professional help."

Laurie's expression was bleak.

"He says he's fine. I think he's afraid to go to a psychologist. He gets angry when I mention it." She put a hand to her face and closed her eyes, trying to hold back her tears. She hated to make it worse for Laurie, but a teardrop trickled past her fingers anyway.

Laurie's eyes filled, too. She took hold of her mother's other hand. "What are we going to do, Mom? How can we help Dad?"

"I wish I knew. Oh, God, I wish I knew!"

"What does Dad think about everything?"

Jean wiped her eyes with a tissue from her pocket. "He acts as if it's a temporary setback. But it's been three years since he resigned as principal, and things are getting steadily worse. He won't even talk to me about how he feels inside." She paused to blow her nose. "He's like a stranger, and I've tried everything to snap him out of it. I just don't know what else to do."

They sat, mother and daughter, in silent pain. Finally a peace settled over them. Jean searched her daughter's face with concern.

"You're about to go to college. You have your future to plan. You shouldn't have this weighing on your mind."

"Don't worry, Mom. I'll be okay. It's you and Dad I'm worried about."

Jean said nothing. Laurie and her father had always enjoyed a special bond. Jean knew that his troubles affected Laurie much more strongly than the girl admitted.

Laurie graduated in the spring of 1974. During high school she had worked with retarded children, and in the fall she would be entering a program for special education at Greenfield Community College in Greenfield, Massachusetts.

In the meantime she looked for a summer job. She found work with a public-service agency, where she met Art DelNegro, a big young man, deep chested, with broad shoulders and a mild disposition. He had graduated from Drury High three years before Laurie did. She knew of him from his high-school days when he'd been a star of the varsity football team.

While attending North Adams State College for a degree in business administration, Art managed a combination sporting-goods, ski-specialty shop owned by his parents. His father, Nicholas DelNegro, had died that year. Nicholas had been head of the science department at Drury High School and taught physics and chemistry. In recent years he had served as vice principal.

Laurie and Art took an immediate liking to each other and

started dating. Besides attending college and helping to run the family business, he tended bar. Laurie found him to be more complex and more dedicated than his jocular, easygoing manner implied.

Home wasn't what it used to be for Laurie, and she spent a lot of time with Art and her friends. In the old days she often declined invitations to go out because staying home was so much fun. Now the reverse was true.

Her mother's efforts to keep the mood light were becoming more strained and transparent. It was plain to Laurie that Jean avoided thinking too much and kept busy with her job at Lamb Printing and with the ongoing tasks of running the household. All their walking on eggshells to avoid awkward moments with Manley had only managed to keep things status quo.

Steven, she knew, tried to be on his best behavior with their dad, but he resented Manley's strange mood shifts and avoided him.

Occasionally Dad looked sad, and Laurie couldn't tell why. He said things that were hard to understand, and sometimes his thoughts would go off on a tangent and not return.

All her friends thought she was exaggerating if she said her father was suffering an emotional collapse. With time, she talked less about her private fears. She, too, kept busy.

One positive aspect of her life was that her family liked Art right away.

At first Art DelNegro listened more than he talked, but after a few dinners at the Tyler home, he began to feel comfortable, and his natural good humor came out.

Art and Manley got along well, but from the first Art wondered about a strange discrepancy he saw in Laurie's father: Before Art met Manley, Laurie had used superlatives when talking about her father. Above all, she emphasized Manley's extraordinary intellect. So upon meeting Manley, Art had expected an articulate, even eloquent, speaker. But, in fact, Manley's speech had strange anomalies: He would use all the correct words, and the thoughts were incisive and the meanings were clear enough, but often the syntax was off; words would be in an illogical or unusual order.

Art had never heard anyone speak in such an odd manner. He never mentioned it to Laurie because she obviously worshiped her father and didn't seem to notice. Art didn't want to sound critical. Besides, it was a subtle thing; he probably wouldn't have noticed it if Laurie hadn't led him to expect someone brilliant.

In mid-September Art resumed his studies at North Adams State, and Laurie went off to Greenfield, where she had rented an off-campus apartment. Tuition at the school was nominal, and Laurie had earned the larger share of her expenses at her summer jobs in the past three years. Still, she planned to find a part-time job while going to classes.

Unfortunately, her special education program was canceled due to lack of enrollment, and Laurie returned home after only two weeks.

She found work at a local printing company and enrolled in art, psychology, and history courses at North Adams State College. She and Art spent every spare moment together.

Art tended bar a few nights a week. Laurie would join him late at night and chat with him when he wasn't busy. One Saturday night in October, Art downed a few scotches after closing. As they sat in the empty restaurant, he looked at Laurie seriously. "Will you marry me?" he asked.

She sat up straight and looked him in the eyes. "How many drinks have you had?"

"It doesn't matter. I know what I'm doing. Will you?"

She studied him skeptically. "Come around tomorrow morning when you're sober. Then we'll see how you feel."

The next morning at 7:30 Art was ringing the Tylers' front bell. He had not slept much. When he was alone with Laurie in the kitchen, he asked again, "Will you marry me?"

"You're crazy. I'm still asleep."

"I love you anyway. Will you marry me?"

After a moment she answered him. "Sure."

Manley's job as rodman ended in December 1974. Jean watched him suffer through the anxiety of being jobless again, silently worrying over the welfare of his family.

He searched diligently for another job, collected unemployment payments, and tried to act confident for her sake.

In February of 1975 he found a job with a local company, Miller Print Works. What kind of a job it was, she didn't know for sure.

Manley described it vaguely: "I mix colored inks for them, and other things."

She asked him why he didn't wait till something better came along. He said he had tried, but that there were no better jobs available. Jean had serious misgivings.

CHAPTER 6

1975–
1976

*N*ineteen seventy-five began, and another winter passed. Manley worked steadily without complaint at Miller Print Works. He was calm but often gloomy. Jean did everything in her power to cheer him, subjugating her own negative thoughts as much as possible. She cooked his favorite dishes, especially the desserts he loved. She babied him more than she ever had before, and he seemed to appreciate it, but his moodiness was becoming chronic.

As the warm months came, she planned more outings with their friends and relatives. Manley seemed most like his old self at family cookouts, yet he maintained a distance in his socializing that had never been evident before. Jean's relatives wondered about Manley's recent job history, but little was said about it openly, and certainly not to Manley.

Jean realized something that she did not want to admit: The role of family provider had been falling to *her* for some time. Manley did not engage in planning and decision making the way he used to. He still took care of the bookkeeping and paid the bills, but gradually Jean had become the decisive one.

Occasionally she still risked an awkward moment by asking Manley about his feelings and the reasons for the changes in his life. His answers were plausible but unsatisfying. Yet Jean clung to them, convincing herself that his recovery was imminent. He said he was fine, and she had little choice but to accept that answer, rather than risking his open hostility by pressing him further.

Steven complained again that Manley had been mean to him, often for trivial reasons or no reason at all. At first she had dismissed this as exaggeration. That was not Manley; he adored his boy. She assumed that Steven was misinterpreting his father's behavior. Now she couldn't help but wonder. They lived in an uncertain and menacing netherworld. She realized that Manley might be creating a private hell for his young son.

As the months passed, Jean was seeing much less of her old friends. She and Manley hardly socialized at all, keeping their hardships to themselves. Laurie spent far less time at home than she used to, so when Jean felt the need to talk to someone, she sought out Angie Potter.

Angie was a dear, funny, irreverent friend from childhood. Since Jean had little confidence driving, Angie offered to take her along to the market on her shopping day. When they had the opportunity, they went out for coffee and conversation.

Angie's husband, Elmer, also knew the Tyler family well. He and Manley shared a love of trout fishing, which had sent them to local streams and rivers. The couples had vacationed together on Cape Cod, where the men and little Steven had enjoyed some saltwater fishing. In years past, the two couples had often dined out and gone dancing with other friends from their social circle.

Jean loved talking to Angie. Her brand of humor thumbed its nose at the tyranny of life. Manley had always fondly called her the "party lady" because she was the spark to many good times.

One Saturday morning the two women took a break from shopping and sat in Angie's car in the parking lot of the local supermarket. Jean talked about the things that had plagued her for so long.

"Our financial situation is a shambles," she told her friend. "His latest job doesn't sound very good. He *can't* be happy about it—mixing colored inks and whatever. Raising two teenagers isn't cheap, as you know."

"You can go broke just feeding them," Angie agreed, "let alone buying them clothes, books . . ." She rolled her eyes.

"Manley and I together don't earn what he used to make alone. What can he be thinking? He worked years to get two degrees—so that he can mix colored inks? He's had four jobs in three years."

"Really?" Angie was puzzled. She had known Manley for more than two decades. "Maybe he's just losing his youthful steam."

"He's changed," Jean said with force. "Radically."

"There's got to be a reason. What does he say?"

"That everything's fine."

"Why won't he talk about it?"

Jean closed her eyes. "I don't know. He's always said that communication is the most important thing in the world. But it's been so long since Manley and I have really talked, I'm beginning to forget what it was like. Maybe this change *is* natural, and I've blown it out of proportion."

Angie thought for a moment. "It sounds like the normal problem that all women have: husbands who don't talk to them. It's too bad that Manley has reverted to form. Now the rest of us wives can't hold him up to our husbands as an example to follow." She chuckled, then soberly added, "Not to make light of your problem . . ."

"No, no, don't be silly," Jean said hastily. She sighed shakily, feeling the onset of tears, and kept silent, hoping that the need to cry would pass.

But Angie knew her friend. She put her arm around Jean's shoulders. "Go ahead and cry, honey. Don't feel shy around me. It's got to come out one way or another."

Sobs swept through Jean. "Sorry, Ang."

Angie hugged her gently, profoundly alarmed at the unexpected force of Jean's emotions.

How good it felt to Jean to have Angie's understanding hug. She had been feeling so alone, so confused.

When Jean had used up two tissues and was blowing her nose again, Angie spoke. "They say you need bad times so you can enjoy the good ones. It's a crock."

"Damn," Jean said softly. "I'm sorry."

"For what? For being human?"

"I hate to burden you. But I just can't figure it out. I feel so stupid."

"Now don't get down on yourself. You're a great wife. You can only do so much." Angie paused, then said, "Time will heal whatever's going on with Manley. Men act strangely when they get into their forties. Sometimes they can be such pains in the butt. We have to be patient with them and occasionally give them a boot in the behind so they can get on with life."

Jean smiled as she wiped her eyes. "It's good to have you to talk to, Angie."

"What are friends for? Manley will talk to you when the time is right. He must have his reasons."

"I can't imagine what they could be. We've been married for twenty-three years—we used to share everything. Now he gets furious when I try to talk about his problems. He hit the ceiling when I suggested that he see a psychologist. He's totally unpredictable— one day he seems like his old self, the next day he doesn't. I never know what to expect—whether he'll be moody and depressed, or be staring at the television for hours, or getting frustrated at the slightest thing. Angie, do you think I'm making too much out of it?''

Angie wanted to ease her friend's mind. "Maybe. Things seem worse when we're in the thick of them. A year from now I'm sure you'll be laughing about it."

"I hope so, Angie. I hope to God you're right."

In the summer of 1976 Manley was laid off his job at Miller Print Works and again collected unemployment benefits. During this hiatus, he decided to go back to teaching. While he looked for a permanent position, he was called to substitute teach in the local schools. He was happy to be with children again, and it showed. But he didn't get hired as a full-time teacher. Jean couldn't understand how that could be; his qualifications were impeccable, his experience and reputation impressive by any standards. Perhaps, she thought, there weren't any openings.

Manley still went to Steven's games and truly enjoyed himself when watching his son play. Steven had pitched the first of his no-hitters in Little League when he was twelve years old. Now thirteen, he pitched four more. And in YMCA basketball, Steven had set two records for high scoring in a game.

Manley was ecstatic over his son's athletic triumphs, but their once-close relationship had disintegrated. They didn't talk about sports the way they used to, in a language all their own. They still would play ball with the neighborhood kids, but their spontaneous exuberance had vanished.

Jean began to notice the friction about which Steven had been telling her. Manley harshly criticized the boy for trivialities. For example, if Steven left his bike in the driveway, Manley would over-react and call his son lazy and inconsiderate. If Steven was a few minutes late for dinner, Manley unleashed a torrent of abusive words. Jean sympathized with Steven but in an attempt to quash the conflict and maintain peace, she tended to support Manley.

Like Jean, Laurie had thought initially that Steven had been to blame for Manley's outbursts. When she lectured her brother to be more circumspect, he reacted explosively. Once the darling of the family, the boy was bearing the brunt of everyone's discontent.

"Dad? Do you know where my baseball glove is?" Steven called from the hall closet.

Manley, clearly annoyed, came in from the den. "What are you doing?"

"Just looking for my glove, Dad. You seen it?"

"*Have* you seen it. Speak proper English."

"Sorry." Steven closed the closet door and went into the kitchen.

Manley opened the closet and looked inside, inspecting the interior. He put his hand up and straightened a box on the top shelf. "Can't you learn to put your things where you can find them? If I didn't watch you, you'd turn this house into a pigsty, like your room." He slammed the door angrily.

It had been a long, disquieting winter. Manley had seemed furious all the time. Steven had to tread with infinite care, but his dad's anger came out of nowhere. Nothing Steven tried to ease the family tension seemed to help.

Manley came in, eyed his son, then went to the refrigerator and took out a carton of milk. He snorted in disapproval as he poured. "Hardly any milk left. See?" He brandished the container and gave Steven a hard look. Then left the room with his glass.

Steven turned away, his face set. Where was that glove? He had searched his room to no avail. The only place he hadn't looked was the basement.

He opened the basement door, flipped on the light, and went downstairs. The large, open space was neat and clean. He went to his father's workbench and looked underneath at the shelves. As he moved aside a large tin of nails, the door opened, and Manley came down the stairs.

"What are you doing? What are you doing, I said!"

Steven backed away from the workbench. "I just wanted to check, Dad," he answered, trying to escape his father's wrath. "I can't find my glove anywhere. I need it."

"That's *your* problem. The workbench is *mine*. Leave it alone, you hear me?" Steven moved away as Manley came all the way downstairs and went to the bench. He turned on the light and inspected the area meticulously. Muttering, he shook his head as he moved the can of nails slightly, to its precise position. "You're no ballplayer. Don't even know where your glove is," he said derisively, with an unkind look over his shoulder at his son. Steven kept very still.

They heard the side door opening upstairs. Laurie and Jean came in.

Manley turned back to the bench and gave it another look. "Stay away."

"I didn't touch anything except—"

"Except! Except!"

The presence of his mother and sister made Steven bold. "Dad, I never take your stuff without asking. I know you don't like it."

"That's right. I don't like it. You . . . sneak! Bugging me about this, bugging me about that—"

Jean came down the stairs, drawn by the voices. "Hi. What are you doing?"

"Steven's fooling with everything."

Jean frowned. "Steven, what've you been up to?"

"Nothing. Just looking for my glove," he said defensively.

Manley said with disgust, "You're no ballplayer. You don't know where your glove is. You're no ballplayer."

Steven's lip quivered with hurt.

"What's the difference?" Jean asked. "He's only a kid."

The boy rose to his own defense. "I'm a good ballplayer, and you know it!"

"Don't you talk to me like that!" Manley exploded.

"Well, you're not telling the truth." Steven looked desperately to his mother for help, but she was staring wide-eyed at her husband, who had taken a threatening step toward their son.

"He's not telling the truth, Mom!"

She whirled toward the boy. "Don't talk like that to your father. You know better than to upset him."

"I'm not!" Steven went to the stairs, away from his father.

"Get out!" Manley yelled.

He pursued Steven, but Jean moved between them. He tried to get past her as he went after the boy. But Steven was already running up the stairs.

"Get back here!" Manley screamed.

"Stop it!" Jean yelled in desperation to both of them. Manley stopped in front of her. "Steven, you apologize to your father this minute!"

Hysteria raised the pitch of Steven's voice, and his eyes filled with tears. "Dad's getting on me for nothing. What did I do?"

Jean said in a level but forceful tone, "He's your father. You apologize this instant."

"I didn't do anything!" He was crying and refused to submit to his parents' unfairness.

Jean was transfixed by her husband's look of rage. "Steven!" she yelled.

But he was rushing into the kitchen, past his sister.

"Why do you always bug Dad and cause trouble?" Laurie demanded. "Can't you leave him alone?"

"Why are you all ganging up on me?" he cried. He grabbed his jacket from a chair in the kitchen, ran to the door, flung it open, and rushed out into the dusk, slamming the door behind him.

In the resounding silence Jean studied her husband and tried to make sense of what she'd just witnessed. "Why are you so mad at him, Manley? What did he do that was so terrible?"

He turned away and checked his workbench. "The sneak!" he muttered. "He shouldn't touch my stuff."

"But he's only a boy," she said to his back. "I don't understand why you were so hard on him."

Manley turned so she could see his profile. "He does it on purpose."

"I'm sure he doesn't intentionally try to bother you. Steven's not like that."

He looked at her then, his eyes unforgiving. "I'm his *father*."

Laurie, concerned, had come down the stairs and stood in the doorway. Manley brushed past them and through the door. Jean answered her daughter's questioning look with a bewildered shrug, then followed her husband upstairs.

Manley had walked into the den and turned on the television. He seemed to want to be alone, so for the time being she let him be, while she and Laurie put the groceries away. Then Jean went into the den. Manley was standing in front of the television but was looking out the window at the gray, blustery twilight. He turned as she approached. His anger was gone, replaced by a lost-boy quality, a humble sadness. He stood awkwardly, as if he couldn't decide what to do with his body.

"What's wrong, dear?" Jean asked.

"Nothing." His eyes strayed to the television.

Something about his posture made her feel terribly sorry for him. She came forward and put a hand on his arm.

"Well, it's over now," she said gently. "These things happen."

He turned to her with a look of self-pity. His eyes were moist. She hugged him while he buried his head in her shoulder. As they clung to each other, Jean didn't dare break the spell by speaking, but her thoughts burned with a new determination.

She knew now that Steven was an innocent victim. How many times in the past had she unjustly decided against him? If only she had known what was really going on! Whatever the cause for Manley's irrational behavior, she was going to take action. *Whatever you're going through, my love, whatever it is you won't tell me, we'll lick it somehow.*

It was after eleven o'clock, and Steven was still out in the night somewhere. Jean had called the homes of all the friends she could think of. None knew where Steven might be. She paced and sat, paced and sat, smoking cigarettes and drinking coffee. Laurie was out with Art. Manley was watching basketball in the den.

She punished herself with self-accusation. She was responsible for the well-being of her family, and she was failing miserably at it. Everything was falling apart, and she was letting it happen. Torn between her husband and her son, she didn't know what to do. Something was wrong with Manley, so she felt that she must protect him at all costs. But that meant neglecting poor Steven.

She gnashed her teeth and sat down again, holding her head in her hands, weeping without sound, so as not to rouse Manley. Finally she put her head down on the table and kept it there for a long time, unable to think.

A few minutes later, the side door opened slowly. Steven finally had come home.

Jean went to him. "I'm so sorry, dear," she said quietly. "It wasn't your fault. I shouldn't have yelled at you."

She noticed his bright-pink coloring from having spent hours in the cold night air. She reached out with worry, but he shrank away from her hand and gave her a hard look. It softened when he noticed her red eyes and evident distress.

"Sit down, Steven. You must be half-starved."

"Yeah," he admitted.

She set chicken and potato salad in front of him and joined him across the table. "Where have you been?"

"All over."

"I was so worried." Jean watched him eat. "Will you forgive me?"

"Yeah," he said.

"Are you going to talk to me?"

"About what?" he asked, his mouth full.

She shook her head and smiled with relief.

"Oh, anything," she said, feeling happier. "Baseball. How you feel. Why you ran out."

"I felt like it. You were all against me."

"We weren't. I just didn't want you upsetting your father."

"Well he upset *me,*" Steven said defiantly.

"I know. He's been really hard on you, hasn't he?"

"Now do you believe me?"

"Yes. Now I believe you." She said it softly so the sound of her voice would not carry. She listened for a moment, but the television was loud in the den.

"Why is Dad always picking on me? I think he hates me sometimes. But he doesn't other times."

She knew it was time for total honesty. She owed that to Steven. "I think something is seriously wrong with your dad, Steven." Jean watched his innocent face helplessly, afraid for him.

"I think so, too."

Her son's words chilled her.

CHAPTER 7

Late 1976–
1977

On the rare occasion that Jean and Manley went out for dinner, they usually accompanied their old friends Angie and Elmer Potter. Angie watched Manley on those occasions for signs of what Jean had described as bizarre behavior. But Angie's impression was that Manley didn't seem so different, except that he was quieter. He didn't joke or laugh the way he used to.

"It varies," Jean told Angie later. "That's why it's *so* confusing. One day he's the man I married, the next he's a moody and apathetic stranger. I never know from day to day."

Angie could commiserate because Elmer had changed after a recent heart attack, but she was taken aback when Jean described the worsening strife between Manley and Steven.

"He must be going through male menopause," Angie responded. "I wouldn't worry too much—Steven will be okay. Manley has been a terrific father to him so far."

"I hope you're right. Since Manley got laid off this time, it's been very tough," Jean said. "I can't understand why he can't get a teaching position."

Angie shrugged. "Maybe he should apply to some other school districts."

"He has. There's been no response."

"Well, there's got to be a reason. It doesn't take a genius to know that Manley is well qualified." She shifted the subject. "What happened at the employment office?"

She was referring to calls Jean had fielded from the Massachusetts Department of Employment, demanding that Manley return four months of unemployment payments. The department representative insisted that Miller Print Works had notified him to return

70

to work, but he hadn't done so. Manley insisted he hadn't heard from his previous employer.

"After a strenuous argument I finally got that straightened out," Jean told Angie. "We won't have to return the money, thank God. But I really had to fight them."

"Didn't Manley fight it, too?"

Jean chewed her lip with a troubled look. "Not really. I was surprised that I had to handle it all alone. There was no way we could pay back the money. Manley pays the bills; he knows the situation. The money was already spent. I had expected him to settle the dispute without my help. But he was . . . I don't know . . . apathetic." She shook her head.

"Can Manley get his old job back?"

"No, it's already been filled."

Angie nodded in sympathy. "What the heck happened?"

"Someone made a mistake somewhere along the line. The department representative accused Manley of trying to get away with something. It makes me angry just to think about it. Does that sound like Manley to you? It bothers him terribly that he doesn't have a job."

"Don't worry. You've had a run of bad luck, but he'll be working again before you know it."

"I don't even want to think about it. I exhaust myself when I do. My little salary doesn't go far, and I'm just taking life one month at a time."

Angie sat quietly, absorbing the information.

"He and Steven are like two boys battling each other," Jean continued. "How can I scold a grown man?"

"I do it all the time," Angie quipped.

But Jean squeezed her eyes closed, trying to find some inner calm. Too often she felt like a leaf carried along on a torrent of confusion. Then, with a grim look, she said, "I'll be honest, Angie. Sometimes I think I can't take it anymore. There are days I'd like to walk out the door and not look back." *There,* she thought, relieved. *I've said it.*

"Join the club. It's only natural, Jean."

"Please don't mention this to anyone."

"Of course not. Do you talk about it with anyone else? Your relatives?"

"No. There's such a stigma attached to mental illness. I don't want the whole town to know about it. I'm protecting him."

"Fine. But who protects *you?*"

Jean allowed herself a brief laugh. "My kids."

A month later Manley was able to find employment through his aunt Charlotte, the sister of Manley's deceased mother. A widow, Charlotte lived in North Adams with her daughter Diane, who was handicapped with cerebral palsy. Charlotte worked mornings for an organization that prepared meals for the elderly poor.

She knew Manley was looking for a job, so she told him about a position she'd heard of in North Adams at a school affiliated with NOBARC, the Northern Berkshire Association for Retarded Citizens. The job entailed teaching woodworking and other crafts to retarded adults. He applied for the position immediately, and the director of the center was charmed by Manley. Within a week he was working.

Some of the spring came back into his step, and some of his old confidence returned. Because he was teaching again, Jean felt new hope.

Steven Tyler had always been an A student, so when he brought home his first C toward the end of eighth grade, Jean was surprised. Manley, who had been finding fault with Steven for trivial things, now turned to criticizing his schoolwork.

Steven's love for his father was tested daily. The boy had learned to defuse many potential blowups and to slip away when Manley's mood turned sour. Unfortunately, dealing with his father was not always as simple as merely avoiding him; Manley's erratic and unpredictable behavior occasionally included the warm intimacy he and his son had once shared on a daily basis. Good-natured horseplay was still apt to occur, especially when they were throwing a ball around in the backyard or playing an occasional organized game with neighborhood kids. When Manley displayed love toward Steven, the boy responded unreservedly. When that love was shut off, Steven was doubly hurt.

One day in late spring Steven, almost fourteen years old, came home from school and found his father in the backyard, readying his vegetable garden for planting.

"Hi, Dad. Want to have a catch?"

Manley nodded but turned back to his garden.

As Steven approached, he thought his father looked tired. Manley was leaning on a hoe, staring doubtfully at a little patch of dirt surrounded by a fence of chicken wire to keep out rodents. The area had a small gate that Manley had made.

"What are you doing?" Steven stopped beside him and stared at the dirt, too. "You planning the garden, Dad?"

Manley turned a vacant stare on his son. "I'm making plans," he answered enigmatically.

"You going to plant broccoli again?"

"I don't know."

"How about tomatoes? Or corn would be great."

Manley sighed wearily. "No. There's not enough room."

"Do you want me to help? We can make a diagram of where everything's going to go."

"I don't need help. I can do it fine by myself. You don't know about gardening."

Steven was undaunted. "I can figure it out. It's not that hard, is it?"

"You're too young. Why don't you do your homework?"

"I already did it."

Manley looked at him skeptically. "When?"

"On the bus. It was easy. I had to read a story and do some math problems. Want to see?"

"No. I don't." Manley's voice had lowered to a menacing pitch. He walked around to the other side of the garden plot. Steven followed.

Manley scowled at him. "Get away from me."

Steven hesitated, looking warily at his father, but took a step closer. "Dad, what is it? Why are you angry?"

Manley's face turned livid. He said nothing as he retreated from the boy's attentions.

"I'm just trying to help."

Manley whirled in a sudden explosion of anger, took hold of his son by his pants and shirt, lifted him sideways, and heaved him away.

Steven landed hard on his side, eight feet away, half in a pile of rocks by the split-rail fence. He lay still, staring at the sky, stunned and disbelieving. He looked over at his father, who was glaring at him with wild eyes.

"Now do you understand me?" Manley asked calmly, as if he'd made some logical point in a philosophical discussion.

In a daze Steven got himself up. His lip and his elbow hurt. He had a hard time focusing through his tears. Without saying anything, he limped away.

73

The youngster stumbled to the road and kept walking. He didn't cry for long; the tears gave way to shock, as if he were outside himself, observing.

When he came to a small bridge, he slid down the embankment to a stream, then sat and stared at the water. He felt strangely older than he'd been only a half hour before. Even his hunched shoulders had a look of age and defeat. Who was this abusive impostor posing as his father?

Steven got himself out from under the bridge and walked in the direction of his house. His mind was assailed by the constantly unanswered questions: *What's wrong with Dad? Why does he hate me?*

Steven passed his home with no intention of going inside. It stood like a hollow symbol of life as it used to be—a cozy center of fun and camaraderie, of delicious aromas of his mother's cooking. Now nothing moved in the darkened windows. He quickly walked down the center of the road, past neighbors' residences to Brian Lynch's house.

Brian was twenty-four, the older brother Steven never had. A skilled emergency-room medical technician at Berkshire Medical Center in Pittsfield, he lived in the basement of his parents' house. Steven was always welcome to visit. They had fun together, just as Steven used to have with his father. Brian liked the boy and would take him four-wheeling off the road in the woods or to run his hunting dogs. Brian also liked to build old flintlocks from kits, and Steven sometimes helped.

Brian's silver pickup truck was in the driveway, so Steven went around to the back and knocked on his friend's private entrance. Brian opened the door and grinned. "Hey, buddy. C'mon in." He was barefoot and wore blue jeans and a green T-shirt. His hair was wet, and he held a towel in his hand.

Steven moved inside and closed the door behind him.

"So what's happening, Steve?"

"Nothing." Steven sat on the couch and looked at the guns on the far wall.

"How come you're not playing ball?"

"I don't feel like it."

Brian looked at him carefully. "What's the matter? You look down in the dumps."

"Yeah," Steven agreed vaguely. "My father and I had a fight."

"What about?"

"I don't even know," Steven said bitterly.

Brian was startled by his young friend's animosity.

"He was just looking at his garden," Steven continued, "and got mad at me."

Brian's brow wrinkled in disbelief as he sat down. "And?" He leaned forward, giving Steven his full attention.

"And he threw me. Like I was a bag of garbage."

"You're kidding me. Manley wouldn't do anything like that."

"He did," Steven insisted petulantly. His look challenged Brian to call him a liar.

"Then what?"

"I left."

"That's it?"

"Yeah. I walked around and came over here." Steven was sorry he had mentioned it. He could hardly believe it himself; how could he expect anyone else to accept it?

"Did he hurt you?" Brian added solicitously.

"Nah." To get out of further explaining, he said, "Dad probably didn't mean it." He felt safe with Brian but shuddered again with the terror he had felt when he hit the ground after being thrown.

Brian took the boy into North Adams for a root beer, and Steven had brightened a little. On the way home, Brian swerved off the main route and drove to a place where the dirt road widened and straightened, with fields on both sides. He stopped the truck.

"Want to drive?" he asked Steven.

"Huh?"

"Hell, I knew how to drive when *I* was thirteen." He turned off the engine, got out, and came around to Steven's side. "Shove over. You're the driver."

Steven slid behind the wheel. Brian showed him how to start the truck and explained about the clutch and shifting gears. Soon Steven had the vehicle rolling along in first gear. Shifting to second was an easier task.

Steven forgot his misery. It was thrilling to be in control of a powerful machine. Brian laughed with him, glad the boy's bad mood had passed.

On the way home he thanked Brian for the driving lesson.

"No sweat, Steve. A little more practice and you'll have it. When it's time to get your license, it'll be a breeze."

Steven would have liked to stay with his friend, but he knew Brian would be going out that night. Alone again, Steven, depressed, walked in the direction of his house. He was elated at having driven Brian's truck, but his encounter with his father was a constant undercurrent.

When he got home, there was a light in the kitchen window. His mom was home. Should he tell her that his father was doing more than just criticizing and venting anger on him; now he was violent? What if he'd landed differently on the rocks or against the fence? Bones could have broken. Just thinking about it made his knees weak.

He walked past his house to the end of the street, where it met Mountainview Road. A car passed him, with hands waving from within—Laurie and Art. Their arrival brought a feeling of security. He waved back, then followed them to his house. Art had been a football player. He and Steven liked each other. As with Brian, Steven had gravitated to Art as a role model while his own father's importance receded. Already Art had protected him from older neighborhood bullies.

Steven opened the side door to the kitchen. His mother was at the stove talking to Laurie and Art, who sat at the table.

"Where've you been, Steven?" his mother asked. "Your father had no idea where you went."

"I was over Brian's. We went for a ride." He sat at the table, close to the window in the corner.

"You didn't spoil your appetite, I hope."

"Nope. I just had a soda. Where's Dad?"

"Downstairs," Laurie replied.

"What's he doing?"

His mother answered. "He's working on that bookshelf he started last month." She gave no indication that anything was amiss.

Footsteps could be heard coming up the cellar stairs, and Steven waited tensely. Manley walked in.

"Hi, Manley. What are you up to?" Art asked.

"Oh, you know. . . ." He moved with easy grace, his posture as straight as an arrow.

Steven watched his father sullenly.

"Steven was with Brian the whole time," Jean told Manley. "They went for a drive."

"Oh." Manley looked at Steven mildly. "We wondered."

"Sorry." Steven was dumbfounded. *Could he have forgotten?*

The meal was pleasant, with lots of joking and verbal sparring between Laurie and Art. Steven watched his father warily but saw no sign of residual anger or remorse. *No one knows,* he mused, perplexed.

He decided not to tell his mother about it, partly because he was afraid of what might happen if she confronted his father and partly because she might think he was exaggerating. He was going to have to deal with this alone.

Steven started classes at Drury High School in the fall of 1977. The new building was far bigger than his previous school, and the student body was ten times that of Clarksburg's. As a freshman he found himself among impersonal teachers, being viewed with condescension by big, manlike junior and senior boys and girls who were budding women.

A year before he had been one of the best-known students in his school; now the bewildering crowds made him feel invisible. Due to the changes in his father, his outlook on life was darker, more brooding, and he didn't make new friends as easily as he used to.

In the uncertainty of change both outside and inside him, at home and at school, Steven's instinct was to withdraw. His pleasure in life was replaced by erratic moodiness. His feelings of dread peaked when he returned home at day's end, caught up in the constant vigilance of dealing with "the problem."

He didn't belong to the same world as his peers anymore.

He tried out for teams, but he didn't connect with his coaches. They were indifferent to him as a person and cared only about his athletic performance. If his enthusiasm flagged, they'd heap scorn upon him. He, in turn, would not exert any effort for them. He couldn't concentrate. As he failed to live up to expectations, adults turned away from him; and he, in turn, judged them harshly. The classroom became a place to sit and waste time. He slid by on the quickness of his mind, retaining enough of what he heard in class to get by.

He stayed at home as little as possible, spending a lot of time at Brian's. Steven didn't talk much about his homelife to Brian because he didn't want to seem like a complainer. He had to be strong and deal with things on his own. His mother and sister were keeping his father's behavior a secret, so he followed their lead.

Manley's job teaching handcrafts to retarded adults ended abruptly. To the chagrin of the school's management, he seemed as mentally unfocused as those he had been hired to teach. He was unable to supervise activities and was forgetful to the point of embarrassment. He was let go.

Once again financial woes took hold of Jean. She didn't know precisely why Manley was fired; he had told her, "They don't need me anymore."

She had a pretty good idea, however: His memory had been getting faulty over the years. He constantly forgot small details: buying the correct items at the store, picking up Laurie from a friend's house, keeping appointments with dentists and doctors, or bringing his car in to a mechanic. Sometimes she would repeatedly ask him to do something, and he would deny that she had asked any such thing. Thus she could guess fairly accurately that he would have difficulty conducting organized activities with retarded adults.

Once again he looked for work. Her cousin Bob MacGowan, a manager for the Cambridge Wire Company, used his influence to get Manley a job at the factory, winding cable onto spools.

After a few days, Bob received complaints from a foreman that Manley was unable to do the work. Bob told the foreman to give Manley time to learn the job, but when he received a second complaint a week later, Bob went to the job site. It was inconceivable to him that a man as highly intelligent as Manley Tyler could not roll cable. The machine that did the work was rudimentary; a child could operate it. Perhaps the foreman had taken a dislike to Manley?. . .

But after observing Manley at the machine, Bob had no choice but to conclude that the former educator really was incompetent. He'd been hearing family gossip to the effect that Manley was having difficulty keeping a job, but this was hard for him to believe. Manley seemed sound of body and mind . . . though a little vague in his speech and far short of the sparkling personality Bob had known all his life. He was forced to let Manley go.

Yet again Manley hunted for a position. He told Jean about interviews he had with managers and businesspeople. "They have all the people they need" or "They'll let me know soon about a position" were typical statements he came home with. Jean didn't question him too closely about gaps of logic in his accounts.

She knew that his self-esteem was far lower than it had ever been, so she avoided contradicting or interrogating him. She kept the peace at all costs.

Homelife, due to Jean's efforts, maintained a semblance of normalcy. Manley drove to and from job interviews and dropped Jean off and picked her up at her workplace. He puttered around his workbench in the basement, building bookshelves and cabinets, as well as pursuing his years-long effort to panel the family-room walls with pine boards. He mowed the lawn. And when he wasn't watching a game on television, he read.

His reading had changed from nonfiction books, especially about history, to magazines such as *National Geographic* and *Sports Illustrated*.

Manley finally found another job with a small company that Jean had never heard of. It sounded like the simplest job imaginable: painting tents. She didn't voice her misgivings to her husband. *Painting tents? What kind of job is that? Is that the best he can do?*

A few weeks later Jean received a true shock when she spoke to Jim Foster, husband of her friend Barbara. Jim was a member of the North Adams Board of Education.

Wanting to satisfy her curiosity, Jean had asked Barbara if Jim could shed light on why Manley had been unable to find work as a teacher.

Jim Foster called her on the telephone. He seemed embarrassed, and he beat around the bush before finally revealing, "Jean, Manley would have been hired in a minute. But the truth is he couldn't fill out the application form properly."

"Oh, come *on*, Jim," she said with a laugh. "You can't be serious."

After all, Manley was extremely proficient at language; he was something of a scholar of American history and had even toyed with the idea of writing a book.

"Really, Jean. I wouldn't kid about it," Jim said apologetically. "He could barely fill out a third of the information. The woman who interviewed him that day tried to get him to complete it, but he couldn't. What little he did write on the form was in a childish scrawl. His name and address were there, plus his age, sex, and phone number; but almost nothing was written in the spaces provided for job history—no dates or any other information."

"I can't believe I'm hearing this," was all Jean could manage.

Jim waited for her to digest the news, then added with sympathy, "Believe me, if there was any doubt about it, he would be teaching now. *I* would have insisted on it. But the facts couldn't be ignored. I can get you the application if you want to look at it. I'm sure it's still on file."

"But he did fine when he was subbing, didn't he?" Jean protested.

"That's true. But we just couldn't ignore this. I don't know what it means, but it indicates that something is wrong. Do you have any ideas?"

"Manley insists he's fine, but to be honest, he's been having some kind of problem." She didn't want to go into it further. "Thank you for letting me know, Jim. I appreciate it."

She hung up the phone stiffly and sat paralyzed in her chair. Memories carried her through a tangle of events. She thought about the day her father died, when Manley couldn't remember his boss's name or the phone number at his job. She also remembered what Bob MacGowan had said about Manley's inability to do a simple job at the cable factory. He'd been working far beneath his ability and still couldn't keep a job.

Another puzzle piece slid into place: A year before, Manley had taken a trip by himself to visit family in Maine. When he got back, he told her that while trying to get to the interstate he had accidentally driven onto an exit ramp and ended up with three lanes of high-speed traffic coming straight at him. He'd quickly pulled off to the side, but it had been a dangerous error. Not being much of a driver herself, Jean had chalked it up to a normal lapse of attention. Now she wondered. And she wondered whether the misunderstanding with the Massachusetts Department of Employment really had been Manley's fault. And there were other questions about his recent job history, his chronic forgetfulness, and his inappropriate anger.

A palpable fear closed around her. Manley's transformation had been deceptively and insidiously slow. Over the years the unpredictability of his behavior allowed her to feel reassured when he acted normal. She'd been avoiding reality for a long time, explaining away or ignoring the countless little clues, making excuses for her husband. What was she really facing?

Alone in her kitchen she wept.

She carried the unfolding awareness within her for days, debating whether or not she should broach the subject of the teaching-job application with him. *Will it make any difference?* Her gut feeling was that it wouldn't. Their talks about his deficiencies had only saddened and angered him, provoking denial.

Instead she gently suggested, yet again, that seeking therapy might be helpful.

"No!" His wall of anger was impervious. "I don't need a psychiatrist. I'm fine!"

On the verge of tears, Jean dropped the subject. She gritted her teeth and grasped at anything for comfort. She always wanted to believe him; there was sanctuary for her in his adamant denials of a serious problem.

But there must be an explanation that she hadn't thought of. She couldn't shake the feeling that it might be emotional. After all, his personality changes were the most noticeable symptoms since his days as school principal.

She knew for a certainty that the responsibility for taking action rested on her shoulders. For a long time Laurie and Steven, taking a cue from her, had minimized Manley's problems to neighbors, family, and friends. Jean hadn't had much contact with the neighbors since she'd begun working; but even to the aunts, uncles, and cousins on both sides of the family who phoned now and then, she said nothing about the day-to-day heartbreak. Her strategy had been to keep the secret within the household; that way, if and when Manley snapped out of it and returned to normal, he wouldn't have the reputation of having had mental problems.

She did seek outside help in one place: That week she called Father Lafayette "Fay" Sprague, a dear friend of the family's and the priest at St. John's Episcopal Church in downtown North Adams. She described a little about their problems and asked if he would talk to Manley in an attempt to convince him to see a psychologist. Fay Sprague agreed to try.

Jean got Manley to go alone to the church by telling him that Father wanted to talk to him. But two hours later, Manley hadn't returned home. Jean called the rectory, and Fay told her of a brief but explosive conversation with Manley.

"We started to talk in a friendly way," the priest said, "but when I mentioned the various problems you were having and that I thought it might be helpful for him to see a psychiatrist, well, he got really angry. He jumped right out of his chair, Jean. He told me to mind my own business, then he stormed out."

Jean hung up the phone, profoundly disappointed. Again she was left alone to deal with the growing chaos in her family.

Two more hours passed before Manley came home. Jean asked him how his meeting with Fay Sprague had gone.

"Can you imagine? He told me to go to a psychiatrist! What nerve!"

Jean felt his accusing eyes on her. "Manley, don't you think we *do* have some serious problems?" she asked meekly.

"I'm not crazy! I don't need a psychiatrist!"

Very softly she asked "How long is this going to go on?"

"It's not that bad. I have a job again." He was proud of his menial job.

She wanted to ask: Whatever happened to your goals, your dreams? Why can't you fill out a simple job application? But she remained silent. How did he view what was going on? Was he keeping secrets from her to protect her, as she was hiding things from the community to protect him?

Manley dismissed the subject and made a sandwich while she sat smoking cigarette after cigarette.

CHAPTER 8

1978

*D*r. William Everett was originally from Larchmont, New York. He'd attended Williams College, Williamstown, Massachusetts, then received his medical training at Columbia University College of Physicians and Surgeons in New York City. After a fellowship in neurology at Yale University, residencies in various hospitals, and a stint as a specialist in internal medicine for the Air Force in Japan, Dr. Everett had returned to Williamstown to join a group clinic. He became chairman of the Department of Medicine as well as director of the coronary care unit and chief of electrocardiography for North Adams Regional Hospital.

In June of 1978 Manley went to Dr. Everett because of a tingling sensation in his stomach and legs. During the examination Manley complained, "I don't know, Doctor, I don't . . . can't . . . do things anymore. A problem with my nerves. Sometimes I can't remember things." The anguish in Manley's voice was unmistakable. "Can't even take care of my own stupid life."

Dr. Everett asked for details and learned where Manley was working. He suspected that Manley might be breathing toxic paint fumes, which could account for the tingling and the evident depression. But he wondered why his patient, who had been a bright, promising teacher and principal and an extremely likable man, had been working at such an unlikely series of odd jobs. Why had Manley abandoned education?

Dr. Everett recalled that Manley had voiced other unusual complaints in the past:

In 1971 Manley had described a warmth and numbness of his right arm and leg, which had persisted for a month. His coordination had been fine, and the symptoms didn't seem exercise related. . . .

83

In 1974 Manley had suffered chronic pain on the right side of his head and blurred or distorted vision in his right eye. Dr. Everett had done a biopsy on Manley's right temporal artery to see if inflammation of that artery could be causing the symptoms. The biopsy had proved normal. An ophthalmologist had examined Manley and thought that his discomfort might be related to sinusitis. Later it was discovered that an abscessed tooth was the cause. Once the last upper molar on his right side was removed, the pain and blurring vision stopped. . . .

In 1975 Manley had complained again of heat in his legs, along with itching and vague chest pains. Dr. Everett, finding no physical cause, thought the symptoms might have been due to work-related stress. . . .

In 1976 Manley seemed to have aching and lameness in his arms, which worsened at the end of the day. . . .

Dr. Everett prescribed Valium to calm Manley, then suggested he take some time to rest. He also advised Manley not to drink alcohol and to return for a more complete exam in a few months.

Manley's job painting tents continued well into 1978. The business was small, with five unenthusiastic employees who looked upon their job as temporary, since it paid poorly and offered a dismal environment—constantly dirty, with the smell of paint and solvents permeating everything.

The workers' opinion of Manley was that he wasn't too bright, and he displayed a dignity out of proportion to his status. This made him a target of frequent jibes. Usually he would ignore their insults, but sometimes he would respond with a threatening look.

He went to work dutifully every workday, in spite of the demeaning experience it often proved to be.

One day, Ray Maynard, an ex-student of Manley's, came in to check on the progress of two tents he had ordered for his private catering business. Ray had been in Manley's eighth-grade class.

Now Ray had come to speak with the manager about an order. The workers were in the large warehouse just beyond the office door. Ray could hear their chatter, and they seemed to be having fun picking on an older worker in coveralls. Ray thought he heard the name Manley, and his curiosity was piqued.

When he finished his business with the manager, Ray asked for and received permission to look in on the employees.

"Manley!" their foreman, a heavy-set young man, said loudly, sneering. "Bring me a can of red and a four-inch brush." He winked to the others, who were watching. "If you don't know which is a four-inch brush, there's a tape measure in the toolbox." Laughter rang out among the employees.

Ray went over to Manley, who was doing as he had been told. The young man recognized his former teacher but experienced a moment of disorientation seeing him in work clothes.

"Mr. Tyler? . . ."

Manley turned to him. At first his expression was puzzled, but then recognition dawned.

"You may not remember me, Mr. Tyler. I'm Ray Maynard. You were my eighth-grade teacher back in 1966."

A smile split Manley's face. "Raymond? You're a grown man! Last time I saw you . . ." He paused, trying to recall.

"Was at Clarksburg School," Ray assisted. "You were principal, and I had just graduated." There were snickers from the other side of the room, which Ray ignored and Manley didn't seem to hear. They shook hands warmly.

"It's good to see you, Raymond. You've grown into a fine young man."

"Yeah, thanks to you, Mr. Tyler. You looked out for me when I needed it. Remember?" In those days he'd been shunted around from one relative to another after the sudden death of his parents, never staying with one family for more than a year.

"You were always fighting, but you had a good heart. I remember."

Ray smiled with affection. "How are you, Mr. Tyler?" He looked around him. "What are you doing here?"

"This is where I work," Manley said blandly. "What do you do now, Raymond?"

"I've got a catering business, which is doing well. My wife and I just had our second child."

"I'm sure you're a good father," Manley said gravely. He looked around as if trying to remember something.

Ray felt saddened. The Manley Tyler he remembered had been like a beacon of light, a benevolent force to the students lucky enough to come under his influence. He seemed older and smaller now.

"Hey, Manley," the foreman called nastily. "Do I have to wait all day?"

Manley turned to him. "What was it you wanted?" he asked.

The foreman rolled his eyes dramatically, drawing more laughter from his workers.

"Forget it, Manley. You'd probably forget on your way over here anyway." The foreman gave Ray Maynard a scornful look.

Ray noticed, and it raised his hackles. When, with exaggerated disgust, the foreman walked across the room to get the brush and paint himself, Ray stepped in front of him. "I'd appreciate it if you showed this man some respect," he said in a deliberately lowered tone.

The foreman sneered. "Who? Manley?"

"It's Mister Tyler to you," Ray said.

The foreman smiled smugly. "*We* don't call him mister."

Ray wanted to punch the man in the face, but he managed to contain his rage. "When I'm around, you'll call him *Mister* Tyler, or you'll answer to me."

The foreman backed up a step. "Hey, I didn't mean nothing. If he's your friend, he's your friend." He raised his hands in capitulation. "Just kidding around. Sorry."

Ray said to Manley, "Good to see you, Mr. Tyler. If anyone gives you any trouble, let me know. I'll straighten it out *quick*." He shot a challenging look around the room. Everyone looked away. Then he waved at Manley, who was smiling.

"Bye, Raymond," Manley said.

"Bye, Mr. Tyler. Take care."

The happy event of the year was Laurie and Art's wedding. Art received his bachelor's degree in business administration and now felt ready to start a family. The ceremony was to be held at Saint John's Episcopal Church in North Adams, with a reception at the Elks Club.

As father of the bride, Manley had to give Laurie away. During the rehearsal he couldn't seem to get his part correct, although what he had to do was not difficult: He was to walk slowly down the aisle with his daughter; then, when they got to the front of the church, he had to lift the veil from her face and say that he gave his daughter to be married. Finally he would take his seat beside Jean in the front left pew.

During the rehearsal Laurie attributed his forgetfulness to nerves. She needed to cue him when to begin the slow walk from the back of the church. When they got to the front, he stopped awkwardly, with a blank expression on his face. Laurie patiently reminded him what to do. Repeating it, he again seemed unable to do it quite right, but everyone was satisfied that the ceremony would proceed without serious mishap—they could guide him through.

The wedding took place on Saturday, April 1, at eleven o'clock in the morning, with Father Fay Sprague officiating. Manley performed his part without incident.

Since Jean could barely afford the expense of a wedding, Art and Laurie offered to pay for half of it, and Jean accepted gratefully. A guest list of about eighty relatives and friends had grown to almost one hundred fifty. Still, the list was kept smaller than Jean would have preferred. The families and friends became acquainted, and merriment ruled the day.

Manley was the lone exception to the revelry. He was rather distant and shy, much different from the Manley everyone knew. To Jean's surprise he rarely left his seat, except to dance. One of his partners was Jean's talkative, energetic aunt Marion. She and her husband, Bob Henderson, had known Manley for over three decades.

"Are you enjoying the party, Manley?" she asked as they circled across the floor.

He nodded with a faint smile.

"Laurie looks just beautiful," Marion continued. "And her new husband is a fine-looking man. I hear he's got a degree in business. Do you know what he is going to do now?"

Manley looked at her, confused. "What?"

"I said, what does Laurie's new husband plan to do now?"

Manley slowed his moving feet and thought about the question. "What do you mean?"

"You know: What kind of job is he going to get? Is he going to continue with the sporting-goods store?"

Manley looked crestfallen. "I don't know. I think so."

Marion changed the subject. "I remember you at your wedding. You and Jean were a lovely couple. Still are, for that matter." She looked at him slyly. "What a handsome devil you were."

As the song ended, Manley looked at her and said apologetically, "I'm sorry—what's your name again?"

She laughed in surprise, taking it as a joke. "Oh, you comedian, Manley."

But Manley was serious.

Manley's good moments were signs of hope to Jean, but the negative episodes became more frequent. She was often moved to pity at his obvious unhappiness and felt afraid for the future. What would happen next?

During this time, Jean found she was losing all authority over Steven. Being occupied full-time with her job didn't help, but she also allowed him extra leeway, hopeful that this might counterbalance the worsening emotional beating he was taking from his father. She didn't have the heart to be as strict as she knew she should be.

In any way she could, she tried to compensate. She gave Steven as much attention as was possible in her busy daily schedule and tried to be as honest with him as she could . . . and hoped for the best. By guile and artifice Jean did her best to shield him from Manley, warning him to keep his distance when his father was in a bad mood or heading off ugly incidents between father and son before they got out of control. Her method was to interrupt and divert the conversation, or to tell Steven to leave the room, or try to convince Manley, in a calm way, that Steven didn't deserve his ire. Sometimes her intervention was successful; sometimes it was not.

Steven didn't have to do anything specific to be rebuked by his father. The boy's presence alone could set Manley off. Steven, reacting with righteous indignation, defended himself and made things worse; then he'd have to leave the house before violence erupted. It was a nightmare for Jean to love two people who were constantly at loggerheads.

Steven was confused by these divergent parental attitudes. He sometimes imagined that he was as unlovable as his father indicated. At other times he angrily fled to spend time with Brian Lynch, who gave Steven the approval he needed.

Steven looked for meaningful connections with other adults as well, but his teachers and coaches rarely showed him any real warmth or interest. He had developed a cocky defensiveness that kept people at a distance. No adults in the school system saw beyond his deceptively uncaring attitude.

Steven's school performance had reached a new low; it was not uncommon to see Ds on his report card. Jean knew it was due to their family life falling apart, but no amount of talking seemed to make any difference. Most disturbing to her was that he didn't seem to care. He called his teachers "jerks" and even disliked his coaches. He referred to school as a prison, where teachers were jail keepers and where students were inmates.

Steven's quick wit and good looks made him attractive to the opposite sex, and he had a succession of relationships but never stayed with one girlfriend for long. As soon as a closeness began to develop, he would break it off. The scorned girl's disgruntlement would circulate in the gossip network of the school, setting him more outside the mainstream.

For his mother's sake Steven avoided getting into serious trouble. But, increasingly, he got into fights. He never fought on school grounds—again, so his mother wouldn't find out. His adversaries learned that he wouldn't fight on school property, and some took advantage of it. Many who taunted him in school avoided him outside. One youth, trying to provoke Steven into a fight in the hall, spit in his face. Steven wiped the spittle off and walked away.

Off school property, however, he fought with and beat some of his antagonists. His battles served as a valve to release his pent-up rage. His ferocity enabled him to vanquish larger boys than himself, but his victories only made him a target for older, tougher boys. Steven didn't care. He was getting used to the role of victimized outsider.

One Saturday early in the summer Jean brought in the mail and went through the envelopes one by one. Paying the bills was Manley's responsibility, but since she had a few free moments, she began opening them. She found a bill from a medical organization—it was four months overdue. In bold red letters it said that unless the balance was paid, a collection agency would be hired.

Jarred from the shock, she opened all the envelopes. Three other bills were overdue. She couldn't understand it—Manley had always been methodical in his bookkeeping.

When he came home, she asked him why he hadn't paid the bills. He answered innocently: "I don't like them."

She couldn't believe her ears. "You don't *like* them? That's it? *That's* your reason?"

"Yes."

During the next few days Jean investigated the rest of their financial affairs. A rude awakening was in store for her: Manley had allowed his life insurance policy to lapse. For once she raised her voice in angry rebuke.

"How could you do such a thing!" she yelled. "The bills *have* to be paid! We've paid premiums on that policy for fifteen years!"

The sheepish look on his face stopped her tirade. He was close to tears.

In a quieter tone of voice she declared, "I'm going to pay the bills from now on. You don't have to do it anymore."

He shot her a suspicious look.

"What's the matter?" she asked.

"*I* take care of the money," he said.

"Do you think I'm going to steal it? It's my money, too." She couldn't believe they were having this conversation.

"We don't have enough money, Jean." His voice sounded fearful.

"You think I don't know that? Our combined salaries don't come close to what you used to make." As soon the words escaped her lips, she regretted saying them.

Manley was genuinely distressed. "We're going down the tubes. Not enough money. What are we going to do?"

"Do?" She laughed hoarsely, uncomfortably. "Like we always did in the old days. We'll throw the bills up in the air, and the ones that land on edge, we'll pay."

He didn't understand. It was an old joke, going back to their early years of marriage, but he'd evidently forgotten it.

Serious again, she pressed her point. "Look, Manley, *I'd* better take care of the bills from now on. You'll get us into trouble if you're not careful." She didn't know what else to say. She was *not* going to allow him control of the checkbook any longer.

Finally he nodded in agreement. He didn't seem to realize the gravity of the situation, and warning bells sounded in her mind. She felt like an impotent fool. Her future was degenerating into something grim and joyless. *I'm blind as well as stupid,* she berated herself. *How could I not see that this was happening?*

That week she called the insurance company and tried to reinstate the lapsed policy, but they said it was too late. They were sorry.

For the first time Jean was beginning to doubt her own view of life. Her upbringing had not prepared her for chaos and despair. She had barely known an unhappy moment till her father had died when she was thirty-eight.

What happened to living happily ever after? she wondered. *Our vows included sickness, but also health; I took him for better or worse—but it's only been getting worse.*

Jean formed a habit of buying an occasional bottle of wine. She would drink a glassful in the kitchen after work and sometimes one later on before bed. It helped her to fall asleep and numbed her when she needed to be numb . . . which was getting to be often.

The evening after she discovered that Manley had been mishandling the family finances, she drank two glasses of wine in quick succession. Her brain was spinning, and she sank into all-too-familiar helplessness and despair. *It's my fault. I had no idea that Manley was so unreliable. I'm in charge now, and I've let us all down. What's wrong with me? Sweet Mother of God! If Manley can be this irresponsible with money, what else is he capable of?*

Emotions overwhelmed her, and she gave in to wrenching tears, sobbing into her arm, which rested on the kitchen table. "I've tried *so* hard all my life, and this is what it comes to. I can't stand it anymore!" She wept in loud, self-pitying moans, surrendering to an excess that she never would have allowed herself had anyone else been in the house. After a while it subsided.

She stared across the kitchen at the empty, irrelevant house—a home they had carefully planned for, working and saving till they could afford to build it. Now it was just space that a disintegrating family slept in, and fought in, even hated in.

She and Manley were only in their forties. They should have been enjoying life, dining out, partying with their friends, and dancing. But she rarely saw people socially; she had become a prisoner in her own life, isolated and wretchedly alone, hiding the truth from everyone.

Manley was taking a long walk. Steven was out, too, probably over at Brian's house—these days she wasn't sure what Steven did. She was losing control of everything: Her husband was a stranger, and her son was, also. At least Laurie was safe, happily married to a good man. A few more tears slid down Jean's face.

She heard the side door open and looked up to see Steven, flushed from the chill air. She straightened in the chair and wiped her eyes, embarrassed to be found like this. Then she realized that Steven had probably suffered similar moments, poor kid.

He looked at her carefully. "What's wrong, Mom?"

She wiped her eyes one last time. "What isn't wrong?" she asked almost humorously, surprising herself with sudden boldness. It was time to be bold. She motioned to her son. "Sit awhile. Don't mind me. I'm allowed to cry occasionally."

Steven sat across from her. His face was filled with concern. "What were you crying about, Mom?"

"About your father. About the fact that your father hasn't been paying the bills on time and doesn't seem to care. And about *you*, Steven? Are you okay? We never talk anymore."

He looked uncomfortable. "I'm fine, Mom."

"No you're not."

He answered her with silence.

91

She reached out and touched his hand. "Something's been happening to your father for a long time, but I haven't wanted to admit it. I thought hiding it would help, somehow. But it doesn't."

Steven nodded.

"We're going through tough times—that's obvious—but I don't want this to ruin your future. You have to carry on and make the best of it. . . ." She trailed off, realizing that she was also talking about herself. "Sometimes things happen that are out of our control, and there's not much we can do but make the best of them. Please try—if not for yourself, then for me."

"Okay, Mom. Where's Dad?"

"Walking." She looked worriedly out the window as if she could see through the darkness to wherever Manley was at this moment.

"Mom." He stopped, and Jean thought he wasn't going to say anything else, but then he continued. "I don't want you to worry. I'll help you as much as I can."

For Steven that was a lot. "Thanks," she said with a smile. "You're a good kid. Don't think I don't appreciate it."

It seemed to Jean that Manley was looking sadder as the days passed. He virtually forced himself to get up every morning to go to work. He'd spoken very little about his job, but she could tell he wasn't happy. Some days he seemed despondent. At breakfast one day she asked him why he looked so miserable, and he answered, "I can't stand it. I hate going there."

But not knowing what else to do, she let the days slide by and immersed herself in day-to-day details, using them as a distraction to keep from thinking too much.

In mid-July Manley and she had just finished breakfast and were preparing for work. She brushed her hair in the bathroom and returned to their bedroom. Manley was sitting motionless on the bed facing away from her. She walked around to his side. He was staring straight ahead through tears that were streaming down his face.

She rushed to him, alarmed, and sat on the bed. "What is it, dear?"

He sobbed, then finally said, "I can't do it. I just can't take it anymore, Jean."

"What? Your job?"

He nodded and held his head in his hands. "I just can't take it anymore," he repeated pathetically.

She put her arms around him and rocked him like a child. Tears brimmed in her eyes, too.

Her beloved husband was in trouble, real trouble. She had waited for years for the problem to go away; she'd wanted to believe him when he said he could take care of things himself. But here he was, weeping helplessly, because he couldn't face going to a job he hated. What malevolent force could bring a proud, strong man to his knees at the prime of his life?

"You don't have to go, Manley. If it's that bad, you certainly don't have to go." She stood up and got one of his handkerchiefs from his night table. She returned and wiped his face gently. "What is it, dear? How do you feel?"

But he just shook his head.

"I'm going to call Dr. Everett. There must be something we can do to help you." She expected him to object, but he didn't.

Handing him the handkerchief, she told him to blow his nose. He obeyed. "Manley, lie down. C'mon." She helped him remove his jacket. He lay back with a sigh. "I'm sorry," he said. "I just can't do it anymore. I tried, I tried. . . ." He started to cry again.

She sat on the edge of the bed and stroked his head. "Anything that needs to be done, we'll do it together, my darling. We'll get help. Lie still and rest. I'm going to call Dr. Everett."

"You're so good," he whispered through his tears.

She went into the kitchen to use the phone. Manley had always visited Bill Everett on his own, but Jean hadn't seen the doctor in years. She talked to the office secretary and made an appointment for that afternoon.

When she called Lamb's, they were agreeable about letting her take the day off. Next she called the tent company and told them her husband was ill and wouldn't be coming in.

All morning she and Manley relaxed, talking and listening to music on the radio. He had calmed down, relieved that he didn't have to go to work.

Jean went alone to Williamstown. For the first time she felt she was taking some positive action. She told Dr. Everett about the morning, then launched into the long list of Manley's unexplained behavior. She described her husband's personality deterioration, the irrational friction with Steven, depressions, mood swings, and memory lapses, and Manley's inability to fill out a simple job application.

"I want him in the hospital immediately," Dr. Everett said. "I want to do a thorough exam and some tests to find out what we're dealing with. He needs to be under constant observation."

"I don't know if I can get him to go, Dr. Everett." Jean looked worried. "He's been so opposed to seeing a psychologist, I don't know how he'll react."

"Tell him that I insist on it, Jean. This is a serious matter."

Determination replaced the worry on Jean's face. "All right. One way or another I'll get him there."

Jean had expected a fight, but when she told Manley that Dr. Everett insisted that he go into the hospital for testing, he offered no resistance at all. Dr. Everett admitted him to the North Adams Regional Hospital that very evening.

Part
II

CHAPTER 9

Late 1978

$\mathcal{W}$hen Jay Ellis was seventeen, his father had died when the cancer in his lungs spread to the brain. It had made a deep and painful impression on him. He had decided on neurology because he wanted to study how the brain worked and why it would sometimes fail.

Years later, Dr. Jay Ellis followed his dream and received post-doctoral training in neurology at the Albert Einstein College of Medicine in New York City from 1973 to 1977. At Einstein College he participated in researching many clinical cases of Alzheimer's disease and other dementing illnesses and learned from a foremost authority on the subject, Dr. Robert Katzman, head of the Department of Neurology there.

Alzheimer's disease was all but unheard of, even by most physicians, in the 1970s. Victims suffering from it were lumped under the general term of *senile dementia,* which was widely but wrongly thought to be caused by hardening of the arteries impeding the flow of blood to the brain. It was the condition thought of for ages as senility, an inevitable deterioration due to old age. Modern medicine had yet to discover why some of the elderly enjoyed undiminished mental ability during their long lives while others deteriorated rapidly into dementia.

Robert Katzman was a pioneer in research into Alzheimer's disease. When Jay Ellis studied with him, Dr. Katzman was the national chairman of ADRDA, Alzheimer's Disease and Related Disorders Association, an organization dedicated to furthering research into causes and treatment and efforts to educate and assist caregivers in coping with the disease. It was Dr. Katzman who alerted the medical community in the 1970s that Alzheimer's was the fourth largest killer of adults in the United States after cancer, heart disease, and diabetes.

Dr. Ellis had continued his research studies under Dr. David Drachman, another expert in the field, at the University of Massachusetts. Jay Ellis set up practice in Pittsfield, Massachusetts, at the Berkshire Associates for Neurological Diseases. Dr. Bill Everett of North Adams called him there about Manley Tyler.

Dr. Ellis met Manley Tyler on the day of his weekly visit to the hospital in northern Berkshire County. A young psychiatrist went into the room with him. Their goal was to determine what was ailing the man whose life had come apart.

Dr. Ellis's first impression of Manley was of his attractiveness. When the physicians engaged him in conversation, he spoke spontaneously but was vague in his speech. He seemed befuddled, and the things he said lacked depth.

After the psychiatrist had completed his preliminary tests, Dr. Ellis conducted some of his own, including having Manley calculate simple math problems in his head and asking for an explanation behind abstract ideas in common proverbs such as "Don't cry over spilt milk," or "People in glass houses shouldn't throw stones." Manley performed competently.

Dr. Ellis tested certain physical responses, including one called "snouting." He tapped a spot above Manley's upper lip just under his nose. In a normal adult there would be no response, but in infants less than a year old or in adults with a loss of brain function, an involuntary sucking reaction would occur. Manley's lips reacted. To Dr. Ellis this indicated an organic rather than a psychological cause to the symptoms.

He conferred afterward with the psychiatrist, who agreed that the problem did not seem to be psychological in origin. Manley was to be Dr. Ellis's patient. He planned to meet Jean and conduct further tests.

Manley was released from the hospital after four days. Dr. Ellis had told him not to return to work, pending further developments. Privately he was fairly certain what the diagnosis would be, but it was necessary for Manley to undergo a CAT scan to rule out any other causes of his symptoms.

Manley stayed at home while Jean went to work. They met with the neurologist a week later at his Pittsfield office. Jay Ellis, barely in his thirties, was younger than Jean had expected. He was slim and had dark, sensitive eyes and an extremely soft voice. She found herself leaning forward so she wouldn't miss any of what he was saying. In a general way he explained the testing procedure and what the physicians looked for.

Then, after settling Manley comfortably in the waiting room, he interviewed Jean in a separate room. She described Manley's series of jobs, each a little humbler than the previous one, and detailed their homelife during his slow decline.

Dr. Ellis told her that Manley had a dementing illness but that more time was needed before he could ascertain exactly what type it was. Until then, they would complete more tests and observe Manley's behavior. But, he warned, Manley could no longer hold a job.

"Oh, God . . ." Jean's heart sank. "What are we going to do? We can't live on what I make."

"I know Manley's too young for Medicare," the doctor sympathized, "but you'll be eligible for Social Security Disability after a six-month waiting period."

Six months! It had rolled off his tongue so easily. She stared at him angrily. As a doctor of neurology in this comfortable practice, he obviously didn't have to worry about having enough money to feed *his* family. What meager savings they had left in the bank would soon be gone. She kept silent while her thoughts raged. She was now the sole provider for her family, which was slipping toward abject poverty. If only she hadn't sacrificed her own college education, she might be better able to support her ailing husband and Steven.

On the way home she made light of the situation for her husband's sake, saying that he could now get a much needed rest from the drudgery of working.

Manley seemed more relaxed than he'd been in some time. He was obviously relieved not to have to work anymore. He was almost lighthearted and joked about the future. "Now I'll have time. I'll read my books," he said.

Jean wondered with pity, *What must it have been like for him to work these last years, without a fully functioning mind?* Then, *Why us?*

Thereafter Manley drove Jean to and from work everyday. He stayed at home, doing chores and puttering around.

Jean thought of asking for financial help from relatives, but, typically, she rejected the idea. *We'll get through this on our own.*

We'll keep our problems within our immediate family. Somehow I'll manage.

She brought Manley to Dr. Ellis's office each month for continued neurological tests. Since Manley's mother had died at an early age and had a history of psychological frailty, Dr. Ellis investigated her medical records; he wanted to rule out possible inherited causes. Although he had pretty much settled on Manley's problem being Alzheimer's disease, doubt would remain until he had the CAT scan results. They would rule out any remaining possibilities, such as a brain abnormality or tumor. Due to a problem with the equipment, however, it was not possible to schedule the scan until December.

Shortly before Christmas of 1978 Dr. Ellis finally felt sure of the diagnosis. The scan revealed no brain tumor or other abnormalities.

He met with the Tylers in his office and told them that he was sure, now, that Manley suffered from Alzheimer's disease, a condition of the brain very few people knew about. It was highly unusual but not unheard of for it to occur in someone so young.

"No tests exist that can prove a case of Alzheimer's disease," Dr. Ellis explained. "We can only diagnose this condition through a painstaking process of testing and observation to rule out all other possible causes of the patient's symptoms."

He told them that its cause was unknown and that there was no effective treatment or cure. He advised them to come in for periodic visits. It was necessary to continue to observe Manley over time to make sure of the diagnosis.

Manley had little reaction to the news. He already knew he was ill. More and more, in a childlike way, he seemed to take his lead from Jean on how to feel.

Jean felt relieved rather than saddened. Finally there was a certainty in her life around which she could organize her strategy for the future. Manley wasn't going crazy after all. They didn't have to fight an unknown anymore; their enemy was not some shadowy threat. It had a name: Alzheimer's disease. Named after Alois Alzheimer, a German physician who first described the condition in 1907, the disease has only been seriously researched in the past few years.

Later, in private, Jay told Jean some grim facts: Alzheimer's was irreversible and eventually fatal. It was marked by microscopic tangles and deposits in many of the brain's cells, or neurons, which increased with time, limiting thinking and memory and causing other dementia symptoms such as personality changes, hallucinations, and delusions.

In more advanced stages, even the patients' physical abilities were affected, until they were confined to bed. Finally the brain lost its ability to function at all, and the patients died, usually of pneumonia, heart attack, or some other secondary condition.

"But what can I do for my husband?" Jean asked. "There must be something."

"You can make the quality of Manley's life as pleasant as possible," he told her. "Since we know so little about what causes Alzheimer's, the most we can do is create as stable and happy a homelife for the patient as possible. Let him know that he's loved and well cared for. That's really the best advice I can offer."

Jean ignored the negativity about it. Regardless what doctors said, if it was real, they could fight it. For now it was enough.

She told Laurie and Art and Steven what they were facing. None of them understood the true impact of the news.

"Is he going to get better?" Steven asked.

"Dr. Ellis doesn't think so," Jean answered. "But there's always room for hope."

"He's just going to stay home?" Steven asked.

"Right. We have to be as understanding as possible."

"So that's why Dad has been so different," Laurie said. "He's not having a nervous breakdown. Now the doctors can help us make Dad better again. We can take care of it."

Steven shared the relief of his mother and sister that the uncertainty was over at last. His father didn't hate him; he was just sick. "We can lick it," the boy said. "With all of us helping, we'll get Dad through this. He'll get well again."

Next, Jean told friends and relatives about Dr. Ellis's diagnosis. Her aunts and uncles commiserated but were at a loss about what it really meant. She had no way of expressing the enormity of the problem because she had hidden the full extent of their suffering over the years. Now she felt she could be open about it. The stigma and shame was washed away by the fact that Manley had a disease, and nobody was to blame.

Angie Potter felt a deepening sympathy for Jean. "I feel bad that I made all those jokes about male menopause," she told her friend on the phone. "I had no idea."

"Now don't get serious on me, Angie. If we can't laugh about things, we'll go crazy. You don't know what a help it is having you to talk to."

For the first time in years Jean felt as if she could take a breath: Manley could stay home now; she didn't have to worry about his getting a job. Once he was home and relaxed, he would get better. Sure, they had a problem, but now that they knew what they were fighting, they would beat it.

Jean looked on the past with a different attitude. Now she had an inkling of what Manley must have been going through, struggling valiantly to support his family right up to the end. She felt ashamed that she had raised her voice to him or blamed him for their troubles.

She was committed to following the doctor's advice. *Don't you worry, Manley. I'm going to make you the happiest sick person there ever was. Your struggle is over, my dear. From now on you can just sit back and let us take care of everything for you.*

CHAPTER 10

Winter
1978–1979

The holidays had always been the happiest times for the Tyler family, and Manley had always been a prime instigator of the fun. But Christmastime of 1978 was bittersweet. Now a more passive Manley was flowing along in their fun, following their lead, and not always catching on to the humor of the moment. Having his family around him in a merry mood made him feel good, so there were many pleasant times over the holiday season.

Jean awaited a downturn in Manley's mood after the holidays. For three years she had noticed that a bleakness would come over her husband at that time, and he didn't recover until spring. This year it was similar, although his more leisurely life-style made his mood less severe. He was able to rest whenever he needed to and do whatever pleased him.

Jean, meanwhile, attended to her job responsibilities, and Steven went to school. They didn't shun people anymore as they'd been doing unconsciously for years.

Jean had minimal but amiable contact with her neighbors, and she felt it necessary to inform them of Manley's brain disorder. They would need to understand any behavioral change that might affect them and their property; also, she knew she might need their understanding.

With the exception of her coworkers, Jean spent almost all her time with her immediate family. She saw her friends even less frequently than she had before Manley's diagnosis, although she still saw Angie or, more often, talked to her by phone. For the most part she lived in isolation.

As usual, finances were among Jean's biggest worries. Her and Manley's joint savings were being depleted as they waited for the public assistance to come through. Jean had begun the process by applying for Social Security Disability in September. Later she had received notices to meet with another physician and psychiatrist in Pittsfield. She accompanied Manley, and the necessary tests and examinations were performed.

Dr. Ellis was tracking Manley's progress, meeting with Jean and him every three weeks. He put Manley through the same or similar neurological tests, plus math, verbal, and logic problems.

Manley performed worse with each successive visit, and he complained to Jean whenever they were about to see the doctor. "I'm not going," he said. "I don't want to take those stupid tests."

"You have to, dear. It's for your own good," she responded, and he would obey.

But she told Jay about Manley's resistance. "It is humiliating for him. The tests are demeaning, reminding him what he can't do anymore."

Dr. Ellis could see that his patient's deterioration was steadily progressive. Because this was consistent with Alzheimer's, he concluded that he didn't need to continue testing Manley, since it bothered him so much.

"From now on," he told Jean, "I'll just meet alone with you. You can tell me how he's doing at home. There will be changes—he will get worse—and I want you to keep me up to date. I'll also want to know how you're doing."

Indeed, it did seem that Manley was going downhill much faster since the diagnosis. Jean had no idea what to expect, despite Dr. Ellis's detailed warning. *How much worse can it be?* she wondered. She had already seen the memory loss, personality changes, despondency, confusion, and rage. But she would not give in or give up. Sometimes she deceived herself, feeding an irrational hope. It was always possible that the doctors could be wrong.

Steven and Laurie were united in that same self-deception. As far as they were concerned, there was no question that Manley would recover.

Jean told herself she was preparing for the inevitable, but she refused to consider that a time would come when she could no longer care for Manley. She refused to think about his death.

Jean confided in her employers, and they were very supportive, giving her plenty of freedom to rearrange her schedule around doctor visits. Her relationship with her coworkers at Lamb Printing became increasingly important. She was grateful for their joking and easy camaraderie. There, at least, she had respite from the uncertainty at home.

Jean thanked God when the Social Security Disability payments began late in February 1979. She also received a small monthly stipend to help support Steven, since he was a minor and came under a special provision. It was still not enough to cover all her expenses, but the pressure was eased somewhat.

Jean and Steven worked hard at keeping a lively atmosphere at home. When Manley did something foolish, such as dressing for church on a Saturday morning or missing parts of his beard when he shaved, they would laugh, and Manley would laugh with them.

As the winter wore on, Jean wondered how Manley felt about passing his days alone at home. He vacuumed, washed dishes, straightened the house, and shoveled snow. As he had since Laurie was born, he did the grocery shopping, following Jean's lists. He had his books on the American Indian, Colonial American history, and the Second World War and Hitler's Germany—subjects that had always fascinated him. He also had television and word puzzles, and he puttered for hours at his basement workbench, with the radio blasting show tunes and classical music.

But the long hours spent inside during the cold weather, particularly at night, made him restless. When no other activity held his interest, he began the habit of pacing from room to room. As he walked around he might spot a magazine lying on a table or one of his tools, which would entertain him for a while. Losing interest, he would continue to move again.

As the weeks passed, he started to pace within the confines of one room. Jean could get him to stop only by talking to him; but when she no longer engaged his attention, he would pace again. The constant restless footsteps made her wish for the warm weather when he could be outside more often.

One night Manley's pacing took him out of the house. Steven had seen him leave, and he had run out after him. Jean heard them go and waited for an hour and a half for them to return. Manley looked relaxed when they came back, but Steven looked haggard. He told his mother of a meandering walk with his father, half of which had been through the snowy woods, dimly lit by the half-moon.

The thought of her husband and son walking in the woods at night in the winter sent a shiver down Jean's spine. *What next?* She wondered.

It was nine o'clock on a wintry New England night. When Jean heard the front door click shut, she got up from a chair in the den to see if it was Steven coming in. No one was there. She looked out the living-room window to see Manley walking away. She knew she had to follow him. She rushed to the hall closet for her winter coat, boots, and hat. Her gloves were in the pockets. She quickly went outside.

Her boots crunched on frozen snow, and her breath clouded in front of her face. The air had the crispness of extreme cold, but fortunately there was no wind. She trotted down the black road between the piles of plowed snow in pursuit of her husband.

At the end of the street she looked around and saw a figure to the right, at the crossroads. She followed. He walked resolutely but without hurrying. In a few minutes she caught up to him. He was wearing a lightweight summer jacket.

"Manley," she said, panting, as she came abreast of him. "Where are you going, dear?"

He looked at her, displeased. "Leave me alone."

"Honey, it's too cold for a walk. Why don't you come back to the house, and I'll make you some nice cocoa."

"No," he said, quickening his pace.

She struggled to keep up. Again she tried, but he wouldn't look at her. "Where are you going, dear? It's freezing out. You'll catch cold."

"Get away!" He shoved her, sending her stumbling sideways.

"Manley!" she said angrily, hoping to shock him to his senses.

Instead he swatted at her with annoyance. "Get away!"

Furiously he continued, lengthening his strides. She hung back, allowing some distance to separate them. Obviously he was not going to listen to her. All she could do was follow and make certain he didn't get lost or hurt. When a few hundred feet separated them, she resumed walking. He slowed to a reasonable pace when she no longer spoke to him. They followed the road as it curved between white mounds of snow. Beyond, the pine woods were dark and silent.

Manley strode through streets bordered by scattered houses and fields, eventually coming to Route 8, a busy road, and turned right. Jean followed as cars whizzed past on the well-salted artery. Beside them the Hoosac River ran between ice-rimed banks. A mile or so farther on, Manley turned right, crossed a bridge, and headed back into residential streets, which would lead them past Stony-brook Drive, where they lived, completing a large circle.

What are we doing out here? she thought. *This is madness.* After another mile they came to the corner of Stonybrook Drive, but Manley continued straight ahead. *Dear God. Now where is he going?*

She approached him again. "Manley?" she said tentatively. "Are you ready to go home, dear?"

He looked at her in surprise. He had forgotten she was there. "What do you want?" he asked.

"I'm worried about you. I don't want anything to happen to you."

He continued to walk. "I'm okay."

She started to say something more, but he flailed at her, and she withdrew to continue following him. This time when he got to the crossroads he turned left. They eventually entered the main residential area of Clarksburg and wandered through streets crowded with homes and parked cars.

Jean was not surprised at the vigor that kept him going tirelessly, but this aimless trek through the deserted streets brought out the loneliness she usually succeeded in avoiding. Despair enveloped her as salt crunched under her cold feet. Golden light angled toward her from the windows of cozy houses of normal families, doing normal things.

Her heart ached. What were the happy families doing? She could barely remember the normalcy she used to take for granted. What she would give to enjoy a few hours of it! She fantasized about knocking on one of the doors and asking if the owners would let her in for a while. She would sit and listen to a family engaged in ordinary nighttime routines, worrying about jobs and homework and what to wear the next day.

Manley turned up the street that would take them past the Clarksburg Elementary School. They climbed the steep hill—two lone walkers, linked by twenty-seven years of marriage, disconnected by a brain gone awry.

When he got to the school, Manley walked into the driveway. Jean caught up as he stood forlornly in the middle of the parking lot, looking at the dark, hulking building.

She stood close to him, then, after a minute, she said, "I'm cold, Manley, and it's very late. Can we please go home?"

He turned to look at her. She sensed a thaw in his mood, and it gave her the courage to kiss him on the cheek. He liked it, so she slipped her arm through his and held tight. "Aren't you cold, honey?" Jean asked.

"Yes. It's cold." He put an arm around her, still looking at the school.

107

"You led me quite a chase. I wish you wouldn't, but I suppose you have no other way of letting off steam. I understand." She was talking more to soothe him than to communicate with him, but he responded.

"I'm sorry, Jean." He looked at her in a way that seemed a little like his old self. "You're so good, so good." He hugged her tightly.

Closing her eyes, she felt a little of the old thrill. She almost started to cry but stanched the tears for his sake. *I've changed*, she thought. *I have to be in control now. Someone has to be strong.*

"Let's go back, dear."

"All right."

Arm in arm they walked home.

Early
1979

*J*ean's initial hopefulness eroded as the weeks passed. Her vow was still strong to do as much for Manley as was possible. If there could be any improvement, she would make sure he had every opportunity. But instead of improving, Manley worsened. Jean, however, adjusted.

Many previously confusing issues began to make sense. Now that she knew he suffered from mental impairment, the signs of his illness became obvious: awkward moments if he tried to speak at length about one topic, the inability to think of certain words or his use of inappropriate words to fill in a gap; the mixing of words in an absurd syntax.

By making mistakes, Jean learned more about Manley's diminished abilities. He hated any change of plans and would explode into a fury. This caused her to realize that he suffered complete disorientation if his routine didn't go as expected. *It's probably frightening for him,* she thought. She found that he needed and relied on a schedule that was the same every day.

Similarly, unexpected occurrences upset him. If a relative or friend dropped by without warning, Manley might leave the room without talking and pace angrily as Jean or Steven talked to the guest. His agitation would continue until the visitor left.

Unfamiliar places made him uneasy. Because Jean tried to offer him a variety of activities, they sometimes went out to eat with Angie and Elmer or one of their other dear friends. They usually went to Howard Johnson's because it made Manley feel comfortable—he had worked there as a waiter during his student days.

Their old friends made the best of these times with Manley, but Jean could see that they were distressed by seeing him functioning at such a low level. He couldn't participate in any but the simplest dialogue. But he recognized his friends and enjoyed being with them, even if he didn't understand most of the banter.

During this period he began losing or misplacing his possessions and would get in a dither looking for them. Jean and Steven would desperately search the house without knowing exactly what they were looking for. "You know, you know," Manley would say impatiently. "That *thing,* that brown thing. I need it."

Often the object he was looking for was his comb or a handkerchief—he had to have a handkerchief and his little black comb in his back pocket at all times. Jean ended up buying several identical combs so that she could "find" one without turning the house upside down.

Occasionally Manley asked where their daughter was. Jean could tell that he missed her.

"She's married. Remember, dear? She and Art live in their own home."

His mental decline was not a constant downward curve. It fluctuated, sometimes by quite a bit. He might seem at a very low level for days, speaking little or unable to answer questions; then the next day he'd talk clearly and articulately for ten minutes. Jean's hopes would soar at those times, and she'd think: *He is getting better. I knew he would snap out of it once he was relaxed and rested.* But an hour later he would be asking where Laurie was and pacing in the living room.

Manley also had spurts of creativity and intense effort. In his own way he was fighting the erosion of his mind with all his might. Jean and Steven found bits of paper around the house with short aphorisms or phrases written in Manley's hand. They were usually of a philosophical nature. Some were so clever that Jean entertained the brief hope that his mental ability was returning, as in "The world teaches me to learn," or, "Talk to me of your dreams." But others were less meaningful: "I hide the door beside you," or, "I see and walk and I go away."

He was usually very proud of his efforts. Jean and Steven made much of them, praising and talking about them, encouraging him to write more.

He still did some reading, or so he said; but it turned out that he was looking at magazines. He showed Jean one of his *National Geographic* magazines, told her he had been reading it all day, and proudly described situations in the photographs.

He can't read anymore, she thought, and later, when she had a moment to herself, she wept. His intellectuality had been the most interesting part of his life. That was gone now.

She occasionally saw him in the den by the bookshelves, running his hand slowly over the beloved volumes of history, Shakespeare, and biographies. He had a wistful look, as if he remembered being deeply attached to the books but couldn't recall why.

* * *

Manley's incessant pacing was becoming an ordinary activity in the household. It bothered Jean terribly at times, but she could do nothing about it—Manley wouldn't stop if she asked him to. Or he might stop, only to start again, like a caged animal.

She had the distinct impression that he suffered a sense of loss. He wanted to do the things he had always done, and when reminded of his limitations, he was driven to emotional extremes. The nighttime wandering was one way he dealt with it, walking off his energy and sadness mile after mile.

Jean included him in whatever she did, making the activity as easy for him as possible; as long as his participation was not too challenging, he could enjoy himself. On Jean's days off she took him for long walks in the neighborhood, which she herself enjoyed if the weather was good. Or she'd go on trips with him to eat hamburgers and fries, always a favorite activity. In the car she would sing. It broke her heart that he couldn't sing with her, but he obviously liked to listen.

She always had a smile and a hug for her man; even when she felt tired or sad, she hid it from him because he was acutely sensitive to her mood. Fatigue and the crushing sadness of her life often brought her to tears. She learned quickly that she couldn't cry in front of her husband; it would make him moan and cry in sad confusion.

In bed before sleep she would hold him and stroke him like a mother would her child, softly reassuring him. He would return her caresses, holding her, too, and kissing her. He still loved her—she never doubted it. It helped to know that.

Their sex life lessened. Sometimes she could tell he vaguely had the urge but was at a loss about what to do. She would help him.

Food always comforted Manley, so she cooked his favorite dishes and always had sweets for dessert and snacks available to him. She often made a bowl of popcorn to eat in front of the television at night, just as she had done in the old days. She fed him frequently because it quieted him, and as the months passed he gained weight. As often as she could, she took him around to visit relatives and friends. He loved to go to Aunt Grace's house for dinner—he could never get enough of her candied carrots.

She brought Steven's television downstairs into their bedroom so Manley would have something to hold his attention before going to sleep. She was often exhausted after working all day and taking care of him all evening. She would try to get him to bed early, so she might have a chance to read a little while he watched the screen.

One day it became evident how strongly his sense of time was impaired by Alzheimer's disease. She had been in and out of the bedroom for an hour, preparing for her next day at work. Manley had been watching the show "All in the Family," When another show had come on and finished. During a third show he asked, "Where did he go?"

"Who?"

"Him." He looked at her as if she should know whom he was talking about.

She tried to narrow down the mystery identity with questions. "What did he look like?"

"Old and funny."

"Did he have white hair? Was he bald?"

"Yes, white hair."

It occurred to her. "You mean Archie Bunker?"

"Yes. Where did Archie Bunker go?"

"That show is over, Manley. It finished an hour ago."

"Oh."

But he continued to look at the screen expectantly. He was still waiting for Archie Bunker to return from wherever he had gone.

Laurie fought Alzheimer's in her own way. She didn't notice anything out of the ordinary because she did not want to notice. Since she was not living in the same house with her father, it was easier for her to deny the truth. If anyone implied that her dad might not recover, Laurie would become very defensive, even combative.

Steven had his own ideas about Manley. He was determined to get his father back, so he tried to sharpen Manley's mental abilities. If they were playing a board game or card game, Steven would try to make his father exercise his brain: "How many points do you need, Dad?" or "You know how to make rummy, Dad. Three of a kind or a straight. Remember?"

Manley didn't appreciate Steven's good intentions, which called attention to his deficiencies, much as Dr. Ellis's neurological tests had done. He would yell in frustration: "Leave me alone! Leave me be!"

"I'm just trying to help, Dad," Steven would respond. "Don't give up. We can lick this. Remember how you used to train me to get better in sports? Now I'll be your trainer."

But Manley would get livid. "Get away from me!" he'd yell.

And Steven would leave the room, hurt and unable to understand why his dad didn't want his help. But he stubbornly refused to give up. He knew that anything was possible if he tried hard enough. That was something his father had taught him.

Manley's habit of denigrating his son had changed. He no longer criticized Steven verbally; instead he glowered at the boy or pushed him away with an angry shout. If they were out of the house, their relationship usually went smoothly, but in the confines of their home Manley erupted regularly.

One Saturday Manley, Jean, and Steven were watching a televised basketball game in the den. Steven sat in the rocking chair, his eyes glued to the screen.

Manley had been watching his son's rocking for many minutes. He tried to watch the television, but the motion of Steven's rocking distracted him until he finally demanded, "What are you doing?"

"What?" Steven asked, continuing to rock.

"Stop it."

Without taking his eyes from the screen, Steven asked, "Stop what, Dad?"

"I said, stop it," Manley looked at his son with a peculiar fixation.

Steven looked at his father and stopped rocking. The crowd's roar from the television captured Steven's attention, and in a moment he was rocking again.

With sudden swiftness, Manley leapt off the sofa, took hold of Steven's chair, and hurled it and the boy across the room. They landed with a crash.

Jean screamed in horror.

Manley stood glaring at his son. Steven was sprawled on the floor against the far wall, the upturned chair beside him. Jean ran to the boy while keeping a wary eye on her husband. Manley's face was twisted with fury.

"Steven! Are you all right?" She helped him up.

Manley looked at her, then back at Steven, who stayed very still, expecting further violence.

"Manley," she said firmly, "sit down."

She motioned for the boy to leave the room while she distracted her husband. Steven stood in the doorway for a moment, watching his father.

"Relax, Manley," Jean requested. "Sit down, dear."

He was still glaring at his son. "Get out, you!" he yelled. "Get out! Get out!"

Jean turned to look at Steven, but he was gone. A moment later she heard the side door slam.

Manley stomped into the kitchen and stared at the door Steven had just left through. Jean looked at her husband's back for a moment, then, seeing he wasn't going to follow Steven, she retreated into the den, collapsed into a chair, and cradled her head in her hands. A small moan escaped her as she rubbed circles into her forehead with her fingers, as if to banish what had just happened.

Oh, God, oh, God. Where will Steven go? Is he hurt? She felt a wave of rage at her husband. He could have killed his own son!

It had not occurred to her before that Manley could be dangerous. She heard him begin to pace in the kitchen.

Steven ran to the woods and sat on a rock near the ice-encrusted brook. He tried not to cry, but tears wet his face anyway. He hated to be weak. He hated to feel this way. He made no sound, but his throat felt like a knotted rope.

"I hate you," he sobbed, punching his fist repeatedly into the frozen ground. "I hate you. I hate you." Pain seared up his arm. "Good," he said.

Manley left the house more often and wandered aimlessly. Jean and Steven would be alerted that he had just left by the slam of the front or side door. Impatient pacing and muttering would generally precede his leaving, so they would expect it and watch for him to go out. His walks always occurred at night and usually in cold, nasty weather. He walked for at least an hour and often for as long as three or four hours, usually without a coat, hat, or gloves, sometimes in thin-soled bedroom slippers. He seemed impervious to the weather.

Jean and Steven never planned a strategy for following him; their routine evolved from necessity. Each of them understood the need to guard him from harm. It was frightening to imagine what could happen to him alone in the woods at night. It was like letting a toddler roam freely. He had to be followed; that was that.

When he showed signs of getting ready to leave, Steven and Jean alerted each other. Whoever noticed his leaving would tell the other while watching out the window to see which direction Manley took. Meanwhile, the one going out would put on clothes appropriate to the weather and bring some gear for Manley.

At nine-twenty one night Jean Tyler looked up from her book and listened as she lay in bed. Manley hadn't returned to the bedroom, and she couldn't hear him. She got up and put on her robe. He wasn't in the kitchen or the living room. She turned on lights as she looked in each room and left them on. She swiftly searched the rest of the house. Manley wasn't in the den, either. She went back into the hall, opened the door to the basement, and peered down the stairs as she flipped the wall switch.

"Manley?" she whispered, though she didn't know why. She was about to go down the stairs when it hit her: *Oh, God, he's gone out.*

She ran to the front door, opened it, and looked out. A cold wind tugged at her terry-cloth robe. The moon, more than three-quarters full, lit the street with soft bluish light. She saw no one. *He might have been gone for fifteen minutes or more.* she realized.

She called to Steven at the top of her lungs. "I think you're father's gone out!"

He didn't reply, but she heard him putting on his shoes and jacket.

Dark images came to her: Manley lying unconscious in the basement, in a pool of blood, having hit his head in a fall. She went to the basement again, but both rooms were empty. She ran back upstairs.

Steven, fully dressed and ready to go out, met her in the kitchen. He saw his mother's fear. "Did you check the basement?"

"Yes."

He dashed out the side door, then came in again. "The car's still here. I'll try to find him."

"Okay. I'll throw on some clothes and look, too," she said, but Steven was already gone.

Jean dressed quickly. In minutes she was out in the night. It was very damp, windy, and desolate. Steven was nowhere to be seen. She didn't know which direction he had taken. Which way should she go? She walked to the end of the street and looked both ways but saw nothing. Manley almost always went to the crossroads, then chose a direction. When she got to the crossroads, she studied the shadowed distances in all directions.

Where are you, Manley? she wondered. Just picking a direction and walking off into the darkness didn't seem intelligent. Jean decided to go home and make some phone calls. It occurred to her that she could take the car, but she didn't trust herself driving the big Ford LTD, particularly at night.

Seeing the house lights all aglow, she thought for a moment that Manley had returned; but the house was empty. She left the lights on, feeling it might act as a beacon for her missing husband.

Her first call was to her daughter. It was possible that Manley had walked to Laurie's house, which was only two-and-a-half miles away. Laurie answered the phone and said that Manley was not there, but Art and she would come over immediately.

Jean's next phone call was to Angie Potter. Elmer answered the phone. He didn't quite understand the problem at first.

"Elmer," Jean explained, "Manley's mind is not what it was. He might get lost or hurt. Anything could happen."

Elmer grasped her concern. "I'll come over," he offered. "The more of us looking for him, the sooner we'll find him."

Jean hung up the phone and thought for a second. Then she called the Clarksburg police and told the officer her dilemma. The policeman had never heard of Alzheimer's disease. For good measure she phoned the North Adams police.

Then she stood at the open front door, smoked a cigarette, and muttered, "Oh, Manley, Manley, Manley . . . you're going to drive me crazy."

By the end of her cigarette Elmer Potter was driving up. Angie had come, too. She met Jean on the lawn and gave her a hug of encouragement.

"Don't worry," Angie said. "I'm sure he's fine."

Elmer joined them. "Which way do you think he would go?" he asked.

"I haven't the faintest idea, Elmer."

Just then Steven appeared at the end of the street, walking quickly toward them. "Any sign of Dad?" he called.

"No," Jean answered.

"I went the way he did last time, and around. I guess he went another route."

"Elmer's going to help us look."

Another car turned the corner. It was Laurie and Art.

The four of them decided to go out in two cars. Steven went with Art; Laurie went with Elmer. Angie took Jean into the house, where they waited by the phone.

In the kitchen Angie said, "You sit and relax. I'll make some coffee."

"Don't be silly. It's my house. I'll make it."

"Sit," Angie commanded.

Jean obeyed, lowering herself into a chair by the kitchen window that looked out across the back field. She vented her fears. "*I* am responsible for Manley's well-being. But it's so hard keeping track of someone twenty-four hours a day. Each time I think that Manley has settled into a pattern, he does something more bizarre."

"Nothing's going to happen to him. How lost could he get?"

"I don't know. Nothing would surprise me at this point." She envisioned Manley in a ditch, bleeding, with broken bones. Was he in the woods? She prayed not. He would never be found in the woods—not till morning . . .

"You can only do so much, Jean," Angie said. "Take things as they come and hold on to your own sanity."

"Any ideas where he might have gone?" Art asked his brother-in-law as he steered the car along through the dark winter streets.

Steven shook his head.

"What was he wearing?"

"Probably just his sweater. That's what he had on at home."

Art shook his head. "It's about fifty degrees, I think."

They drove carefully and slowly, covering all the local neighborhood. They saw one fellow with a dog. They stopped and asked him if he'd seen a man walking alone, but he had not. Next they went west, in the direction of Williamstown, and passed Clarksburg Elementary School. The car's headlights probed the darkness, but all Steven and Art saw were empty streets and houses lit from within. They talked to a couple of people who were outside but learned nothing.

Elmer and Laurie ended up in North Adams and drove down those streets. Every time they saw someone walking they thought it was Manley.

Laurie had been quiet for a long while, succumbing to a mood of desolation. *Where are you, Daddy?* she agonized. Her mother had been so frightened. Was it so unusual? *Daddy's probably having coffee at the doughnut shop or visiting with some friend. He's probably laughing right now, cozy and warm somewhere, while we roam around looking for him.*

Manley came home on his own at eleven-thirty, with a Clarksburg patrol car not far behind him. He walked in the side door and greeted Jean and Angie as if nothing was wrong.

With relief Jean said, "You went out without telling me, Manley. It makes me worry."

A moment later the doorbell rang. Jean talked to the policeman at the door.

"We spotted him a few blocks from here," he told her gravely. "We followed him to see if he would come home. I thought it might upset him if a police car stopped him."

"Thanks," Jean said sincerely. "That was smart of you. I appreciate it."

When she returned to the kitchen, Angie and Manley were making small talk. Jean looked at her husband. He looked robust from his long hike.

Motioning at the door where the policeman had been, Manley asked in all innocence, "What did he want?"

She shot Angie a weary look, then answered her husband. "They were just asking for donations to the policeman's fund."

Steven and Art pulled in soon after. Steven wanted to know where his father had been and asked him directly.

"I was walking," Manley responded pleasantly. He seemed unaware of the trouble he had caused.

When Laurie and Elmer had returned and they all were leaving, Angie said to Jean, "Get some rest, kiddo. It's been a long day. You look tired."

Jean smiled. "Who, me? Tired?"

Once in bed, Manley fell asleep easily. Jean lay awake, listening to his even breathing and waiting for life to continue.

CHAPTER 12

Late Spring
1979

*M*anley's moods varied over an entire spectrum. Simple happiness was usually accompanied by humming, as when he was engaged in something like sanding a piece of wood or having a catch with Steven. When dark moods gripped him, he would churn with an inner battle, pacing and hitting the walls and furniture with his hands as he passed. If he had to do something he didn't like, such as change his clothes, he would throw a childlike tantrum, raising his voice or hurling something across the room. Most often, however, he just sat and stared at nothing.

He tried a different expression of desperation that spring. One night, after a day of restless pacing and inconsolable brooding, he went upstairs to Steven's bedroom and threw himself against the window. The frame rattled, but nothing broke. He walked back a few feet, then ran and heaved himself against the window again. When it held, Manley cursed and struck at it repeatedly with his arms. As he pounded on the window frame, Steven came running upstairs, with Jean close behind.

They found Manley banging his upper body against the wooden crosspieces. Unintelligible sounds of despair escaped from him.

"What are you doing, Dad?" The boy's voice held a note of hysteria.

Without answering, Manley took a few steps away from the window, then turned and ran at it again. Steven lunged and grabbed Manley from behind, slowing his momentum.

"Dad!" Steven cried, still holding on to him. "Don't! Please!" There were tears in his eyes.

Jean came up behind them and put her hands on her husband's shoulders. "Please, Manley. What are you trying to do?"

119

Leaning against the glass, he sobbed. "I . . . can't . . . stand it! I . . . can't . . . stand it!" Tears ran down his face.

Jean started to cry, too. "I know it's hard for you, you poor dear." She moved in front of him.

He looked past her, then touched his head with his fingers. "Die," he whispered.

"Come downstairs, Manley," Jean urged gently. "I'll cook something nice for you."

He pulled away and moved to the other end of the room. Jean and Steven stood uncertainly, then walked toward him. Manley charged between them and hurled himself at the window again. Steven tackled his father and hung on as they tumbled to the floor.

"No, Dad! I'm not going to let you!"

"Let go! Let go!" he yelled. Manley thrashed around, pitting his larger frame and greater weight against Steven's. But the youth was like a tenacious cat.

"I won't!" Steven held on with all his strength, managing to restrain his father underneath him.

Jean knelt and held Manley's shoulders down, adding her weight to Steven's. She spoke soothingly, trying to calm Manley, who lay on his side with one arm pinned beneath him. He was flailing at Steven with the other, but it was more an expression of despair than anger.

At last their wrestling slowed, and they lay still. After some minutes Manley tried again to free himself, but Steven tightened his grip. The cycle repeated twice more until they all were thoroughly exhausted and lying in a heap on the floor. Their tears had dried. Jean stroked Manley's hair.

He put his hand to his head and said, "This thing . . . this thing in my head . . ."

"I know, my darling," Jean said with a sob. She couldn't get any other words past her constricted throat.

It took almost an hour for Manley to calm down to a point at which Jean believed he wasn't going to try to hurt himself.

When all emotion had faded, they got up and went downstairs. Manley sat down in the den and watched the television as if nothing unusual had transpired.

Jean sat in the kitchen and wept, absently wiping her tears away with soggy tissues.

Steven came in and watched her for a minute.

"Mom? Don't worry. He wasn't really going to do it. He could have gone right through that window if he'd wanted. I think he just doesn't know what else to do. He really doesn't want to kill himself."

But three days later Manley tried it again. As before, it was nighttime, after a restless day. Steven, alerted by the sounds of his father's increasing frustration, saw him make for the stairs and raced after him. Manley had opened the door to what used to be Laurie's bedroom, then crossed the hall and went into Steven's room. He turned and ran through the doorway and across the hall, heading for the window in Laurie's room.

Steven sprinted in pursuit and tackled his father before he reached his destination. The boy pulled Manley onto the bed and held on tightly, lying half on top of his father. Jean came in a moment later and helped to keep Manley down. Steven was sweating and exhausted.

Jean and Steven took turns for a long time talking in soothing tones to subdue Manley. With his far superior strength, Manley could have easily overpowered the teenager and freed himself; but he didn't.

Steven did not feel any anger directed at him. Even after all that had occurred, he believed that his father wouldn't hurt him.

A month later, after listening to Manley pacing fitfully for an hour, Jean heard him pound up the stairs. She followed, expecting more crashing against the window. Instead, her husband stood at the top of the stairs, misery etched on his pained face. She realized that he was going to throw himself down the stairs.

"Manley! Don't do it!" she commanded.

He ignored her. "Jump . . . jump," he said, teetering on the top step.

"You'll just hurt yourself. The stairs are carpeted, Manley. A fall can't kill you."

He seemed not to hear. He leaned forward.

Jean screamed, "No!"

But he threw himself down the stairway, tumbling like an oversized rag doll, thumping heavily. She leapt to where he lay crumpled near the front door.

His eyes were open. "Jean?"

"Oh, God, Manley. Does anything hurt? Can you move?"

After pushing himself up to a sitting position, he rubbed his head and his left elbow. Physically he was fine.

"No good. This thing won't let me. . . ." He was tapping at his head insistently with a finger, pointing to his enemy. "No good, **no** good."

She sat with him on the floor with her arms around him. "You're only human, my darling. You can't help what's happening to you. No one could."

Dr. Jay Ellis had seen many cases of Alzheimer's, but never in one so young. Increasingly, he worried for Jean and the children. Jean told him of the chaos and emotional devastation her family was experiencing. She phoned the neurologist to ask his advice about Manley's suicide attempts.

"Alzheimer's patients usually do not attempt suicide, but it's not unheard of," he told her. "Each person is different. The brain is still a great mystery, and we can't predict what Manley's exact behavior will be like, except that it will get worse."

When Jean made no response, Dr. Ellis continued, "You have to begin thinking about the eventuality of placing Manley in a facility where trained professionals can take care of him."

"Never," she said quietly.

"You're not going to have a choice. I'm sorry. But I can prescribe tranquilizers for when he's at his worst. That may help. We'll have to see."

After a pause he added, "This disease is fatal, Jean. That is a fact you can't escape from. I wouldn't take away all his options."

After hanging up, Jean sat in shock, thinking of the implications of what he said.

After some weeks, however, she began to view the situation differently. *If he has to suffer and die, maybe it's better if death comes quicker.* But she doubted that Manley was capable of killing himself.

Dr. Ellis mulled over the plight of the Tyler family, wishing he could do more for them. That this cruel disease was destroying such a youthful man and his family seemed especially unfair.

The part of Alzheimer's about which he knew the least was the day-to-day devastation of families. Time after time he had observed that the loved ones also became victims. All the ramifications of emotional stress were impossible to comprehend without experiencing caregiving personally. Caregivers wore themselves out, often destroying themselves and others around them. All too often the grim results were divorce, emotional breakdowns, ruined health, even death. He'd heard of caregivers driven to drug or alcohol dependency or even suicide as they watched their loved ones become as helpless as infants.

Laurie Tyler DelNegro was out of the home and spared some of the agonies; Steven Tyler was another matter. What would the slowly unfolding tragedy do to him? The young felt themselves to be immortal, invincible. They didn't believe in disease or death. And, of course, the bulk of the burden was on Manley's wife.

Jean was beginning to face the hard reality that things were not going to improve. She could feel herself changing, preparing for more of the same . . . and worse. A numbness had been growing within her, an anesthetic to the incessant demands of her daily existence. Once active in the church, Jean felt her spiritual faith weakening. *God wouldn't do this,* she thought. *At least no God I want to know.*

From moment to moment she carried on, adapting to her husband's ups and downs. She could never be sure what he felt, and Dr. Ellis couldn't tell her, either. That was beyond present knowledge, even among neurologists at the forefront of Alzheimer's research.

The family's dogs and cats were a great comfort for Manley. They demanded little and responded lovingly. He could sit for long periods petting one of the animals. He enjoyed walking Buttons and Babe and generally preferred the company of animals to people—people were demanding.

Though Manley's brain was functioning far below its normal level, he still perceived people's emotions and attitudes. He had lost the ability to keep up with ordinary conversation, and he became upset if a visitor was loquacious and expected responses. He could tell if someone felt ill at ease with him, and that made *him* uncomfortable.

But Manley continued to have moments of clarity, even insight, when there was a glimpse of his old self. It was as if the brain, which was fading steadily each day, enjoyed brief comebacks, lighting up previously dead connections for a while.

During such blessed moments, Jean could relate to him on a more meaningful level. He might say, "You're good. You're so good," and she would know that he understood that she was trying to do the best for him. His love for her had not died in the same way his brain was dying. And she could love him in return and find the strength for another day.

Manley repeated his suicide attempts at the upstairs windows a few more times. When Jean was the only one home with him, she would gently dissuade him from smashing through the glass.

"Please don't do it, Manley," she would plead, afraid he would cut himself. "It's not far enough off the ground to kill you. You'll just hurt yourself and feel worse."

When Steven was home, he would wrestle with his father and hold on with all his strength until the self-destructive impulse passed. Meanwhile, Jean would help by saying comforting things.

After such episodes the boy would be exhausted physically and emotionally, wearing a look of premature age on his face. It seemed to be as Steven had said: Manley didn't really want to hurtle through the window; but just needed to express his frustration and rage in a futile cry for help.

* * *

Midnight. The silence of the house did nothing to calm Jean's fretting. She sat on a corner of the couch in the den. Her body was so exhausted it felt only a hollow ache. Tears coursed down her cheeks. *There won't be much sleep tonight,* she thought.

Most of the evening Manley had been calm, but at around eleven he'd begun pacing. Soon he was moving from one room to another, picking up decorative objects from shelves and tables, replacing them, and moving on, then doing it all over again when he came back to that room. He didn't notice the objects as he touched them; it was an automatic action, devoid of meaning. He touched whatever he encountered—wall, window, cabinet, chair, or door. He touched a thing briefly, then moved away with no apparent satisfaction.

His movements had become progressively more urgent, and when he came to walls or furniture, he hit them hard with his palm, expressing frustration and impatience. Finally he had thrown open the front door, and she knew he was going to go out. *Not now,* she'd groaned inwardly. *Not right before bed.*

Steven had told her, "I'll go, Mom. I'll follow him."

She hadn't argued. She was very tired. It seemed that she had been tired for years; unfortunately, she was unable to take advantage of the moments of quiet.

The day before, Manley had gone for a walk in the middle of the night. She had gotten up, dressed quickly in semisleep, and followed him out, walking behind him until almost dawn. Now, having worked all day, she was exhausted.

124

The emotional and physical strain of the past eight years was unbearable at times. *Maybe I can relax a bit.* She closed her eyes and prayed. *Please, God, give me rest.*

The quiet was shattered when Steven burst in through the side door, yelling for his mother. He sprinted through the empty kitchen, down the short hall, and into the den, where she rose, heart pounding, to meet him.

"Mom! Dad's at the bridge. I think he wants to jump!"

"Oh, dear God." She grabbed a sweater from the couch and ran past him, out the door and into the chilly night. Steven was on her heels. "Which bridge?" she called over her shoulder.

"At the end of the street, over the creek."

She and Steven raced to the the small bridge. Manley stood stiffly, gripping the rail with both hands and gazing down into the shadows where water slid by nine feet below.

Jean ran to his side. She was cautious as she addressed him. "What are you doing, Manley?"

He pulled violently away from her touch. "No!" he protested, scowling.

She spoke calmly. "You don't need to be out here. Come on home."

"No!" He clutched the rail and rocked back and forth. Jean touched his arm again gently, and he swung around, throwing her back. "No!"

Jean stayed away then.

Steven, rooted with fright, stood on the other side of his father. "No, Dad . . . please don't."

"Christ," Jean said in anguish to herself. Her heart was thumping. Expecting the worst, she pictured her husband moaning in pain as he lay broken and bleeding in the icy stream.

Jean had learned that if she spoke loudly or angrily, Manley became more agitated. She had trained herself to speak quietly, even though her fear was great.

"It's rotten what you have to go through, dear, but is it so bad that you want to die? I try in every way I know to make you happy, Manley. I don't know what else to do. I don't know what you're going through. . . ."

Manley did not look at her, but he stood very still and listened. The absurdity of his trying to kill himself by jumping off this tiny bridge struck her.

"If you want to jump," she told him, "we can't stop you. But you can't possibly kill yourself by jumping. All you'll do is crack your head open or break a leg or an arm. You don't want to hurt yourself, do you?"

He remained silent, still gazing down into the black rushing water.

She continued conversationally, "You might have to go to the hospital, wear a cast, and stay in bed for God knows how long. Is that what you want?"

He looked at her, then looked down again. "No more," he said. He hit the side of his head with the heel of his hand. "No more! No more!"

Pity forced tears into her eyes. "You poor dear. It must be awful. But we're here, and we love you. We'll see it through together, Manley, like we always have." She knew that part of his misery was because he felt worthless and was a burden on her. She knew how he must hate that, in moments when he was aware enough to realize it.

"After twenty-five years of marriage, we know each other inside and out, don't we?" she asked with soft intensity. "You know I'll see this through with you, Manley. Don't you worry, hon. I'll be with you all the way."

She continued to talk quietly, trying to express all the things she imagined he would want to say but couldn't. She rambled, and he listened. When he seemed closer to jumping again, she reiterated that he could break his legs if he persisted.

Almost imperceptibly, his suicidal mood lifted. His despair was expressed in soft weeping, and Jean was able to lead him back to the house. Steven held on to his father's other arm as they walked.

From the corner of her eye she could see Manley and Steven, father and son. No family should have to go through this. This was not what she and Manley had dreamed of for themselves or for their children. This despicable illness had created a web in which they were all trapped. The only thing that kept them going was their unabating love for the man they remembered as having been warmhearted, joyful, and intelligent.

Back at home, with Manley settled down at last, Steven asked her, "Why his *mind*, Mom? Why did that have to be taken from him?" His eyes held a look of suffering well beyond his years. "If they ever tell me I have this disease," he added, "I'll commit suicide."

CHAPTER 13

Summer
1979

For Manley's sake, and determined to help him in every way possible, Jean and Steven fought despair. They worked constantly at making life seem normal, maintaining the "family" camaraderie. Jean joshed her husband with simple humor, and Steven horsed around when the mood was right. They played simple board games or card games—Monopoly or Sorry or Rummy or Go Fish—in the family room in the basement or watched television in the den. Manley could no longer play Scrabble, one of his favorite games, but he could hold cards and move a piece around a board after rolling dice. Soon he would no longer be able to play Go Fish.

As the weather warmed, Steven encouraged his father to join him throwing a ball back and forth outside, which Manley enjoyed. He was still as deft with his hands and as agile as he had always been.

Manley functioned fairly well by himself at home while his wife worked and his son attended school. Any small chore he could complete around the house bolstered his feelings of self-worth; he wanted to be useful. He vacuumed the rugs, though only in the middle. Because he liked to wipe the dishes dry, Jean started washing them in the sink instead of using her dishwasher.

But as time went by, Jean noticed that Manley was putting the dishes away in places other than the cupboard. She was finding other household goods in unlikely places, also. She might find cans of food in the living room or in the clothes closet; dishes were stacked in the basement, while magazines or books might be piled in the refrigerator.

Once, when Steven brought her a package of frozen pork chops he had found in the bathtub, they had laughed so hard their sides ached. Manley had laughed, too, although he had been the "culprit."

When Jean came home from work, she sometimes noticed that pieces of furniture had been moved into illogical arrangements. Chairs, lamps, vases, books, and other odds and ends might end up in a cluster in the middle of the room or all in one corner. Jean could rarely discern any logic in this odd redistribution. Replacing her furnishings became part of her daily routine, but she would never complain or find fault in Manley. In effect, she was letting him know that whatever he did was all right.

Steven, always quick to adapt, also worked to create light moments rather than awkward ones.

Jean observed signs that Manley was losing his grasp of reality, and it made her increasingly fearful for his safety. She'd seen him try to make a sandwich but with poor results, or he would make the sandwich then walk away without eating it. He had started asking questions such as, "Where's bread?" if he wanted to make a sandwich. "Do I take bread out?" he would ask. He wasn't sure about anything anymore. Whatever he tried to do he would ask, "This way?" at each step of the procedure.

After a while she discovered that he wasn't making his lunch as she had thought. He would be ravenous when she arrived home from work. As a result she made his lunches and put them in the refrigerator; but at day's end she found them uneaten. She began to call home at midday and remind her husband to eat. When even that didn't work, she would make sandwiches that wouldn't spoil, such as peanut butter and jelly, and leave them on the counter for him.

There were further clues to his decreased functioning. If Manley buttoned his shirt incorrectly, he wouldn't notice or would make the same mistake again. He often forgot to put on a belt or put it on incorrectly. For someone who had always been fastidious about his clothing, these were unmistakable signs of low capability. Jean's imagination subsequently conjured the many ways he could hurt himself—she feared he might even set the house on fire.

To assist Jean in her task of caring for Manley, Dr. Ellis had prescribed tranquilizers and sedatives for his patient, including Mellaril, Haldol, and Thorazine, to be used as needed. It was Jay's intention to make Manley more manageable in the worst times and to minimize Jean's hardship. Jay had confidence in her judgment: Jean tended to be conservative in the use of the pills; she didn't want to overmedicate Manley and further dull his senses. Her goal was to maximize the quality of his life, not to make things easier for herself, although Dr. Ellis told her often she should minimize her own stress whenever possible. But she didn't want Manley sitting like a zombie all day, or disoriented and hallucinating. She tried to maintain a balance where he could be happiest and the household most harmonious. Often she went for a week or two without giving him any pills.

Since individuals react differently to medication, especially in unpredictable circumstances such as Manley's, Jean had to assess when and how much of a medication was called for at a particular time. Some drugs were to calm her husband; others were to moderate his mood or to help him sleep soundly at night. Luckily Manley was very cooperative about taking his medication.

Jean visited Dr. Ellis once a month for the first eight months of 1979. Then her visits became less frequent, and most of their contact was done via the telephone. She would call during moments of crisis when she needed advice or just to discuss Manley's deterioration. Although Jay did not know a lot about care and management of Alzheimer's patients in the home, he was supportive and helpful and made himself available, which Jean truly appreciated.

Through her confidences, he alone understood what she was facing. He affirmed her plight and assured her that what she was doing was right and proper. Each step of the way he tried to prepare her for the worsening of Manley's symptoms and urged her to look after herself.

"Neglecting your needs will not help Manley," he said, suspecting her tendency to do just that.

He continued to touch upon Manley's eventual placement in the care of professionals. It was inevitable he told her again and again. "It's desirable to be prepared for this step, since it is only a matter of time."

Jean listened but resisted. Her belief was that she and she alone could give Manley the best care. Steven was another story. He plunged into self-destructive rebellion that she felt powerless to counteract. Jean felt wholly inadequate at protecting the fifteen-year-old from their nightmarish homelife. No adolescent should have to follow his father up and down streets and in and out of woods in the middle of the night. Nor should he be the brunt of his father's rage or a witness to his father's suicide attempts.

She wished she could express to Steven the depth of pain she felt for him, but she knew that was impossible. She prayed that someday he would understand. Steven was frequently out late. He drank beer with friends and had taken up smoking as a form of defiance. This was surprising because Steven had hated anyone to smoke around him. He even had a No Smoking sign on his bedroom door in a clear message to his mother, who had always smoked.

Jean feared where his rebellion might lead. His report cards were consistently awful, but he didn't seem to care. She tried to make him see reason, explaining how he was hurting himself. She shed tears, expressed anger, pleaded—in fact, she tried everything she could think of. None of it had any effect on him.

Steven insisted that he could work things out for himself. He refused to confide in her. All he would say is, "Don't worry about me. I can handle it. I'll be all right." Jean wasn't so sure.

Stars twinkled, and a warm breeze blew. Steven had heard the front door open and close. He had alerted his mother, then he had slipped out into the dark after his father. Manley had gone to the end of the street and turned right. At the crossroads he had entered a path that cut across a grassy slope, then disappeared into the woods.

Steven picked up his pace so he wouldn't lose sight of his father. When he walked past the first few trees the darkness of the woods enclosed him in a patchwork of moonlight and thick black shapes. Invisible roots and stones across the path caused him to stumble. The woods at night belonged to predators. He hurried on, wanting to close the gap between his father and him. Manley walked steadily ahead, like a sleepwalker. He never looked behind him, although twigs and leaves crunched loudly under Steven's feet.

Steven was thankful when his father chose the path that led into the open again. In a few minutes they had left the woods and were on a country road.

Steven knew his own role was important; on these weird excursions in the dark he was his father's protector, ready to help if he was in any danger or difficulty. It gave Steven a purpose that he lacked in any other aspect of his life.

He didn't want to hate his father and tried hard not to. Manley was a powerful man, and when he grabbed Steven and used his full strength, it was frightening. To Steven it made his petty fights around school seem like child's play. His mother had repeatedly explained that the disease was doing it, not his father. But it sure was his father's body.

A healthy body and a sick mind, Steven mused.

The road led back into the streets not far from their home. Steven followed his father up the hill and past the school where Manley used to teach. Steven remembered how, in another lifetime, they used to play soccer in the hallway at home, with the kitchen door as one goal and the door to the den as the other. They kicked a balled-up pair of socks over the polished wood floor while his mother and sister yelled like cheerleaders.

Steven had lost sight of his dad. They were in a neighborhood thick with huge trees on both sides of the street. Steven peered frantically ahead for any movement. In a black shadow beneath an old maple he almost bumped into his father.

"Dad." He felt self-conscious.

"Steven?" His mood was pleasant. He seemed happy to see his son. "Nice out."

"Yeah. Sure is."

"I'm walking." His body language invited Steven to join him.

They walked silently together through the pools of light from the street lamps and the glow from lighted thresholds and windows. Steven waited for cues from Manley before speaking. No longer father and son, man and boy, they were rough equals now— he was maturing into manhood, and his father regressing into childhood.

He liked when his father was having a good day, when Manley spoke more intelligibly, without inventing words and leaving thoughts unfinished. It didn't matter that his words sounded as though they came out of a first-grade primer.

As they turned a corner Manley pointed. "Look. See? See? Raccoon." He ran toward it, and Steven followed, but it had disappeared through a row of bushes. "Gone," Manley said. "Looking for food. Smart."

Steven laughed, delighted with how relatively normal this was. "Remember that time when we were camping, Dad, and the raccoons opened our cooler and ate our butter and bacon and everything?"

Manley laughed. Steven wasn't sure if he remembered or not, but it was good to hear him laugh.

Steven glanced at his wristwatch. Tonight they'd been out almost two hours. He was accustomed to the late hours. He could sleep till noon everyday, skipping school if his mother didn't get after him.

"Ready to go back yet, Dad?"

Manley looked around but didn't answer, so Steven rephrased his question. "Tired yet? Want to head home?"

"No. No." Manley lengthened his strides in childish defiance.

Steven shook his head, reached into his pocket, and brought out a pack of cigarettes. He had never smoked in front of his father, but what the hell, he thought. He fell back a few steps and lit the cigarette. When Manley didn't notice, Steven felt a small thrill of getting away with something forbidden.

They passed the boundary of North Adams and entered the village limits of Williamstown. They were about four miles from home. There was a pond around a bend, and Steven got the idea to divert his father's attention, as his mother sometimes did. He picked up a few rocks and ran ahead. Then he stopped by the pond and waited for his father to catch up. As Manley approached, Steven began tossing stones into the water.

"Look how pretty the ripples look," he said, then held out a stone. "Here, Dad. Want to throw one?" Steven avoided making a contest out of the activity, since he knew that could frustrate and anger his father.

Manley stopped and accepted the stone. He felt its rough texture, then, after Steven tossed another one, he threw his. They watched the ripples, then Steven offered another stone and searched the ground for more. Manley threw it and started looking for stones, too.

Steven wondered if his father would stay there all night throwing stones. He flung another stone and muttered to himself, "I wish things were different sometimes. I miss the old days. You and I used to be a team." He hurled the next stone with angry force. "Shit."

"This thing . . ." Manley said.

Steven's head came around.

"This thing in my head . . . won't let me. . . ."

Steven stared.

"Won't let me . . . do what I want . . ." Manley stopped and started again, "Your mother . . ." Words failed him then.

Steven saw his father's eyes glisten with tears. He put an arm over Manley's shoulder. "It's okay, Dad. What can you do?"

Manley hung his head and draped an arm over his son's shoulder. "This thing . . . damn thing in my head," Manley repeated, touching his head with the fingers of both hands. He looked into his son's eyes.

Steven had the impression that his father understood everything but was unable to express it. He dropped the stone in his hand. "What do you say we head home? Aren't you hungry?"

"Yeah," Manley agreed.

On the way to North Adams Steven talked to his father about sports, school, even that he knew how to drive a car. His chatter was easy, and although he didn't expect or get any reaction, it felt good to express his thoughts.

They ended up on the road that passed Clarksburg Elementary School. As they came to the playing field beyond the school, they stopped and threw more rocks for a while, aiming at a trash can. It rang out with a metallic bang a few times before they moved off toward home.

Manley began a project at his workbench in the basement. During the weeks that he concentrated on it, he seemed calmer, more sure of himself. Having a sense of purpose often made a world of difference in his moods.

Manley was building something out of wood, and for weeks Jean and Steven heard him sawing and banging away, with his radio blaring. In past years Manley had made shelves, cabinets, and a table or two, so Laurie and they were curious about this project; but no one was supposed to see it till it was finished.

Finally Manley summoned Jean and Steven to his work area. They walked down the cellar stairs with excited anticipation. Manley led them to the far wall and stood proudly beside his masterpiece.

It was taller and wider than a door, many layers thick but essentially flat, made by nailing thin pine boards of varying widths and lengths together at haphazard angles. It crowded the eight-foot ceiling of the basement. It didn't look like anything, but they had come down to praise it, and praise it they did.

A few days later Steven helped Manley carry it out the cellar hatch and into the backyard, where Manley wanted to display it. As an abstract wood sculpture it looked rather interesting, Jean decided, but she asked Steven to remove it several weeks later. Even though none of the neighbors had complained, it was so odd she didn't want to have to explain what it was.

Manley's big Ford LTD looked beautiful, but when it was raised on a service-station lift, the mechanic told Jean that the frame had serious rust erosion. He advised her to think about getting another car, since he didn't feel this one was safe.

Jean had been thinking about ways to stop Manley from driving, so this was not totally bad news. More and more his driving was a matter of extreme concern. She knew he was a safety hazard to himself as well as to others. It was common for him to make wrong turns. He would find himself on a street he didn't know and feel bewildered. Recently his driving had been limited to dropping Jean off at work and picking her up afterward.

He loved his LTD, and she feared his reaction if she asked him to give up driving it. Buying a different car might make the job easier. She was hesitant about bringing up the subject of buying a different car, but she had no choice.

To her surprise Manley didn't object. She went to a number of dealers, looking for a modestly priced used car, and settled for a Ford Fairmont station wagon. Manley was with her. He did not participate in the transaction other than to say repeatedly, "A lot of money."

He drove the station wagon home. The next morning, however, she told him, "Manley, I think I'll drive myself to work from now on." She braced for an argument, but he merely nodded. *The disease is progressing,* she thought. *Is he glad to relinquish the responsibility of driving?*

Her relief was short-lived. Panic gripped her. Although she'd had a driver's license since 1966, she had hardly used the privilege. The few times when it had been necessary, she had been petrified every second she was behind the wheel. This was yet another unpleasant task she had to face.

I have to get to work, she reminded herself. She slid behind the steering wheel. After many minutes she started the ignition. With her heart pounding, she began the four-mile ride to her job.

The moments when Manley seemed to return to himself were a blessing, brief partings in the clouds of incomprehension. More and more, however, the bizarre was becoming the norm. Manley's speech and behavior resembled those of an insane person.

He would make up words, what his doctors called *neologisms.* And Jean knew that he suffered from delusions. Dr. Ellis warned her that Manley might even hallucinate.

"I'm in trustle for," Manley had said once, then looked at her, expecting a response.

"What do you mean, Manley? I don't understand."

Loud and clear Manley demanded, "Can't abole? Hah?"

Usually, though, Jean understood her husband through his body language and because she knew him so well. He might say: "Glass milk . . . want," which was obvious, as were requests dealing with most of his physical needs.

The greatest difficulty arose when he tried to express ideas and emotions. Jean suspected that he felt and understood far more than he could verbalize. He greatly appreciated her efforts and would say, "You're good," or more typically, "Good, good." He was thanking her or telling her how good she was to him.

Once he had come to her and said, "Hant . . . I want . . . see, I want. . . ." He stopped and shook his head.

"Are you hungry, dear? I can make you a sandwich." That was often it.

"No no no no. The thing . . . and arn can't . . ."

She waited patiently through his struggling silence.

"No. See see see?"

"Is it something you're trying to find?"

"No no no! It! It!" He stamped his foot in disgust.

She shook her head, drawing a total blank. "I'm sorry, Manley. I'm having a hard time understanding."

He stormed away from her, muttering, "Hard time hard time time."

She thought to follow him to try again, but experience had taught her to let it be rather than stir up trouble. If it was not important, he would forget and go on to something else.

"A laugh a minute," she said to herself. He had been inventing words for years actually; strange words would be hidden within sentences that sounded fine otherwise, although his exact meaning was unclear.

As Manley regressed, Jean's worry over Steven intensified. He was more frequently the undeserving target of Manley's abuse, which had turned physical all too often by the end of the summer of 1979. Manley raged at him over the slightest things. In the beginning, Manley's verbal attacks occurred about once a week, but now they were becoming a daily experience. Steven didn't have to do anything to provoke an attack.

The only reason Jean could think of for these spontaneous outbursts was that Steven's presence reminded Manley of what was missing in himself, and it sparked his fury. The boy was quick to sense danger and learned to get out of the way before Manley could get his hands on him.

Steven tried to stay away as much as he could, but he still lived at home. The house was a battleground. Refuge was anywhere outside.

One rainy night Manley was particularly agitated. The weather had been gloomy all day, and he had not been able to settle into any activity. Instead he had paced incessantly, covering every room in the house, much as he did as a prelude to bursting through the front door.

Steven had spent the evening at a friend's house and was driven home because of the pelting rain. As he came in through the side door, his mother sat at her sentry post, the kitchen table. He was about to take off his jacket when Manley came into the kitchen.

"Get him out!" he shouted, his face red with rage. "Get him out! Don't want!"

Steven froze as Jean got to her feet.

"You don't mean that, Manley. Steven didn't do anything. He's soaked, the poor kid."

Manley yelled even louder. "Get him out! My sickness is him! Out of my life!"

Jean stared in horror at her husband, then at her son. Steven's face registered profound hurt as he whirled and ran outside.

Jean leapt to the door. "Steven!" But she caught just a glimpse of him running full speed as he disappeared past the neighbor's house. She felt certain he was crying. She turned back to the kitchen. Manley was gone, but she heard him pacing in the den, muttering, "Out, Out! My house . . ."

She was numb. What would Steven do? Where would he go? *Brian's house,* she decided.

She was still standing, wondering what to do, when Steven came in again. He was dripping wet, his dark hair plastered on his scalp. His eyes were wild.

"Thank God you're back," she breathed. "Your father didn't know what he was—"

"Yeah, right," Steven muttered without looking at her. He passed by quickly, stopped at the entrance to the hallway, and listened for his father. Satisfied Manley was not waiting in ambush, Steven tiptoed into the master bedroom. Jean heard a jingling of her car keys. The boy came out swiftly and passed her, heading for the door.

Jean followed, grabbing his shoulder. "Where are you going?"

"Out." His hand was on the doorknob.

"Please give me the keys. I don't blame you for being angry—

you have every right to be—but you must give me those keys. Now." She kept her voice low, not wanting to make a scene or incite Manley.

"I have no other way to get anywhere, Mom. It's pouring out, and Brian isn't home."

"Steven, you don't know how to drive. You don't have a license."

"I know how to drive," he retorted.

"Since when?"

"For a while. I'm good at it. Nothing will happen. I promise."

Jean lost control. "I can't believe I'm hearing this!" she raged. "You're not insured. You're underage. What if a policeman stops you?"

"Don't worry. I won't do anything stupid." He opened the door.

"Steven, I forbid you to drive that car!"

"What do you want me to do? *Walk* into town?"

"Maybe one of your friends can pick you up. I'll drive you."

"Mom, you hate driving, especially at night. You may not know it, but I can drive better than you."

"I absolutely forbid it!" Her voice had risen.

"I'm going, Mom." He went through the door.

Jean followed him into the rain. "Steven!"

He looked back at her with regret. She was crying, but that didn't stop him. Before he got into the car he said, "I have to, Mom. I have to get out of here. I can't go into the house, and I refuse to walk for miles in the rain."

She considered trying to wrest the keys from him, but she couldn't picture the outcome of the struggle. So she watched helplessly as he started the engine and backed the car out of the driveway.

When the taillights were out of sight, she went back inside, praying that he wouldn't get into an accident. For hours she sat and cried. How could Manley have said such horrible things to Steven, who loved his father despite the abuse and mistreatment?

For the first time she wondered if Steven might consider suicide. She prayed harder than she ever had in her life.

In the early morning hours Jean heard Steven drive the car into the driveway. She had lain in bed beside her sleeping husband for hours. She listened as Steven crept quietly upstairs to his room. She let out a sigh of relief, but sleep didn't come till much later.

Jean had no choice but to face what her husband's illness was doing to her son. Steven had just started his junior year in high school but was hardly attending any of his classes. It was doubtful that he would graduate without retaking courses he had failed. She couldn't watch his life be ruined. For the first time she admitted to herself that placing Manley in an institution might become necessary at some point.

Dr. Ellis was sympathetic to Jean but told her that the strife between Steven and Manley could continue indefinitely. Jean decided to ask her relatives for advice and assistance. She was proud of her self-reliance, but her son's future was at stake.

Aunt Grace, a sunny woman, was Jean's mother's sister. Grace had married the voluble Jim MacGowan, whom everyone called Teet. He and Grace were good-hearted people always willing to help.

When Jean told her uncle about Steven's problems, Teet was visibly moved, and she could see he was surprised by how bad things were. Teet suggested that the family get together to discuss what might be done for Steven. That week he talked to his two sons, Jim Jr. and Bob.

Bob MacGowen offered to have the gathering at his house. He came to visit with Jean privately a day before the family powwow. "I had no idea things were so terrible," he said. "Why didn't you tell us?"

"I didn't want to burden anyone."

He gave her a knowing look. "What do you think family is for? I want you to tell me what's going on from now on. Nobody should have to deal with such a problem alone."

"Amen to that," she agreed.

Jean's aunts, uncles, and cousins gathered in Bob MacGowan's large house to discuss Manley's worsening behavior and what could be done for Steven. It was suggested that the boy would benefit by living away from Manley. Bob volunteered to take Steven in, since he and his fiancée, Cheryl Berry, had plenty of room. Cheryl, a special-education teacher, was eager to help, and Bob had always liked Steven. Bob had known Manley all his life and was familiar with his style of firm leadership. He believed that Cheryl and he might be able to give his second cousin some much-needed structure in his daily life and provide him with a more stable home environment.

They took the next few days to think it over. When asked for his opinion, Steven did not object. *The poor kid has had it,* Jean thought.

Steven wondered how his mother would fare on her own with his father, but he acknowledged it might be easier for her if he wasn't in the house to set his father off. He would only be a few miles away whenever she might need him. He felt sad but relieved as he packed his belongings.

When next Bob MacGowan saw Jean, he voiced another concern: "Are you going to be all right alone in the house with Manley? It might be dangerous for you."

"Don't worry Bob. Manley has never been violent with me—just with Steven."

Everyone expected Steven to do better at school now. He promised to try, but to him, school was meaningless, something to get through.

Bob knew that his cousin had been getting away with too much. It was his aim to help Steven get refocused on his schoolwork. Thus he set down a loose framework of rules for Steven, attempting to re-create the fatherly guidance that had been lacking. Steven was to stay home two nights a week and go with him to the library one evening a week to study. He also assigned certain chores to Steven, notably to help with splitting a load of firewood for the wood stove.

Steven earnestly tried to made a success of the new arrangement. He knew he had moved in with Bob for his own good and to make life a little easier for his parents. He called his mother almost every night to make sure she was all right. But his habits were too firmly established to be changed overnight. He escaped to Brian's house or went out with other friends every chance he had.

CHAPTER 14

Fall
1979

*H*aving her son move out of the house was like a page turning in Jean's life. Although it felt good to have the support of the extended family, her emotions were in conflict. On one hand it was terribly unfair to Steven that he had to move out of his own house; she knew it was the logical thing to do, but as a parent she felt guilty about it. On the other hand, she also felt greatly relieved that he wouldn't be part of the nightmare.

Manley didn't seem to miss his son. Jean had told him that Steven was going away for a few weeks, and Manley hadn't commented. He calmed down somewhat, which was a blessing since she no longer had Steven's help to watch or follow Manley.

Jean spoke to her daughter at least once a day. Laurie avoided the subject of her father's condition except in the most hopeful light, and Jean protected her daughter and eased her fears, tacitly going along with Laurie's continued denial and unrealistic optimism.

She was thankful for Angie Potter, who listened to her problems and helped her to joke about them. To laugh and thumb her nose at Alzheimer's, as awful as it was, helped a great deal. Jean did so when she could, but alone with Manley there were fewer and fewer laughs.

One day in October Angie came up with the idea of having an afternoon together away from Manley, thus giving Jean a little break. She talked to her husband, and Elmer volunteered to watch Manley at the Potters' house while the two women went out.

It was not an easy thing for Elmer to be with his old friend in this sad condition. Considerable time had passed since they'd all been together, and the change in Manley was hard to believe. It shocked Elmer to see how dependent Manley was on Jean now.

140

While she and Angie prepared to leave, Manley would not allow her out of his sight. Jean assured him that she'd be back before too long and that Elmer and he would enjoy themselves.

As soon as the women had gone out the door, Manley went to the front window and watched their car till it was out of sight. Then he roamed the living room and adjoining kitchen, returning regularly to the front window. Elmer turned on the television, per Jean's suggestion.

"What do you like to watch, Manley?" he asked as he flipped through the channels. Manley stared at him, then sat in an easy chair and watched a movie while Elmer thought of the good times they'd spent beside remote mountain streams fishing for trout.

Jean had encouraged Elmer to talk to Manley conversationally even if he didn't understand.

"Remember when we used to fish, Manley?" Elmer asked. "We used to traipse all over these mountains." He gestured out the window at the distant mountains in view. "Some days we brought home a mess of fish. The girls hated to cook them. Remember how they used to get after us? Lord, we had some good times."

But Manley wasn't looking at him. He was staring at the television.

Elmer continued, "I haven't fished much this past year yet. Maybe you and I could go sometime." Elmer became absorbed in his own wandering thoughts. "Did you know that I had a heart attack a couple of years ago, Manley? It scared me, made me look at life differently. I realized that it wasn't worth the energy to worry about most things. Better to relax and look at life with a little humor. It doesn't do any good to feel bad about things you can't change."

Manley turned to look at him with some interest. For a minute Elmer thought he understood.

"You're still here. You still remember your old friend, don't you, Manley?"

Manley responded to Elmer's smile with one of his own. It made Elmer feel better.

"Where's Jean?" Manley asked, suddenly rising from his chair.

"She and Angie went out for a little while. Remember?"

Manley started to pace again, with particular interest in the front window, looking outside each time he passed it. He said, "Jean's boyfriend. She . . . boyfriend. She left."

Elmer was shocked that Manley seemed to be accusing Jean of

leaving him for another man. "You've got to be kidding, Manley. She went out with Angie, remember?"

"Party lady."

Elmer laughed. "Right! That's my Angie." It heartened him that there was still a vestige of the old Manley in there somewhere.

"Boyfriend," Manley said. "Left me."

"No, Manley. No way. Jean would never do that."

Manley paced, peering suspiciously out the window every other minute. "Where's Jean? Where's Jean? Where's Jean?" The anguish in his voice said more than his short phrases.

"They'll be back before too long," Elmer said, trying to mask his own sinking feelings. *Poor Jean. Now I know why she needs to get out.*

"Left me."

Elmer tried to get Manley's mind off the fixation on Jean, but Manley couldn't be distracted.

"Want to go for a walk, Manley? It's nice outside."

"Yes, walk." Elmer got Manley's coat, helped him put it on, then he donned his own jacket. They went out the front door. It was a mild October day.

Manley stopped at the top of the front stairs. Elmer went down the five concrete steps and waited at the bottom.

"Coming, Manley? Let's go." But Manley drew back, afraid.

Elmer was puzzled.

"Don't you want to go for a walk, Manley?"

"Yes." But he didn't budge.

"If you want to go for a walk, you'll have to come down the stairs," Elmer told him. "There's no other way."

"No."

Elmer came back up and tried to coax Manley down, but he refused. When Elmer took his arm, Manley got a panicky look that stopped his friend. There was nothing to do but go back inside. Elmer opened the door and went in. Manley followed but started pacing again. Elmer sat and watched him as he went about, touching things without interest. Elmer was tired already. *How does Jean do it?* he wondered.

Manley opened the front door and went out to the stairs again and stood there. Elmer joined him.

"Walk," Manley said.

"Yeah, sure. I'm ready when you are."

But Manley would not come down the steps.

"C'mon, buddy, you can do it."

"No." Manley went back inside again.

Elmer shook his head and sighed. *This could go on forever.* He watched Manley's pacing and listened to more paranoid speculation on Jean's whereabouts. It hurt Elmer to listen to him.

"Left me. I'm bad," he said.

"Don't say that, Manley. You're a fine person, and you know it. Jean loves you."

"No. Left me, left me, left me."

"She's with Angie. You know how the boys go out together? Well, the girls have to get out, too. She'll be back soon. Don't worry."

Manley went out yet again to the stairs. Elmer could tell he wanted to walk, but the stairs bothered him for some reason. He looked down and couldn't move.

"I know you want to walk, Manley. All you have to do is go down five steps. It's easy. They're just like your stairs at home, except there are two extra ones. Come on. You can do it."

Manley actually started to go down the first one, but he retracted his foot at the last minute, like a pathetic child immobilized by fear. Then unexpectedly he said, "Hold my hand."

Elmer looked at him. "Hold your hand? If I hold your hand, you'll come down the steps?"

"Hold my hand," Manley repeated.

Elmer shrugged. "Okay. That's easy. Ready?"

He took hold of Manley's hand, and the two men went down the steps like a father and child. Finally they were able to have a good long walk around the neighborhood. Manley still expressed fear that Jean had left him for someone else, and Elmer did his best to allay those delusions.

When they returned to the Potter residence, Manley soon became even more agitated about Jean's absence. Elmer was at his wit's end watching his old friend roam from room to room, hitting the backs of chairs and tabletops. He decided to try to contact Jean on the telephone, thinking that the sound of her voice might pacify Manley.

After a few phone calls, Elmer located Jean and Angie.

Elmer explained the situation, then Jean talked to her husband. Elmer watched Manley grow calmer. After they hung up, Manley remained reassured for a while and watched the television. But by the time Jean and Angie returned an hour later, he was pacing again. It seemed to Elmer that Manley's life was suspended when Jean wasn't with him.

Having moved in with Bob and Cheryl, Steven had to take a new bus to and from the high school. Their neighborhood was near one of the tougher sections of North Adams, and while waiting for the bus, Steven found himself surrounded by a gang of older boys who taunted him. One fellow was egged on to pick a fight with Steven and finally incited Steven to hit back. With others kicking at him from all sides, Steven was no match for the larger boy. From then on he avoided the bus. But even walking, he was forced to sneak through the neighborhood to get to Bob and Cheryl's home.

He intended to stay in the house two evenings a week, but he didn't keep track and escaped with friends every chance he got, sometimes just to smoke cigarettes. He went to the library with Bob once a week. While Bob did research for graduate courses he was taking, Steven tried to do his own schoolwork, though often he just faked it for Bob's benefit.

Bob encouraged Steven to discuss his problems or feelings, but he was no more successful than Jean had been. Steven insisted he "had things under control."

Bob and Jean had discussed Steven's school problems. Because Bob and his brother had been outstanding students, Jean thought his influence might be helpful when talking to Steven's teachers. He agreed to accompany her to meetings at the high school.

First Jean met with Steven's guidance counselor and asked for help in salvaging the boy's education. The counselor agreed to call a meeting for all of Steven's teachers. Bob came with her at the appointed time, but only one teacher showed up.

Jean explained the enormity of the family's stresses and asked the teacher if he and Steven's other instructors would monitor the boy's behavior. She requested special reports every few weeks on how Steven was performing in the classroom, plus any other pertinent information, so they might gain a foothold in his academic recovery.

The teacher agreed, but he was the only instructor to give Jean a report. It was clear that the other educators didn't care. Their indifference stunned her. She was further outraged when the one teacher involved sent her a note saying: "Steven has to grow up."

You fool, she thought bitterly. *The problem is he's growing up too fast.* It was a supreme irony to her that Steven was the son of an educator truly worthy of the title. Manley would have gotten some action out of them if he were well.

If one of these teachers had half the commitment to their students that Manley used to have, she thought, *what a difference it would make for Steven. If these are educators, then God help the children.*

CHAPTER 15

Late Fall 1979

$\mathcal{J}$n Steven's absence, Manley's anger occasionally turned on Jean. He had a child's thinking processes and self-centered instincts, along with the impatience, fears, and irrationality. Even when he couldn't express in words what he felt, she would know he was angry because he would pull away from her embraces and rebuff her kisses or sweet talk with a scowl. His reasons were seldom clear and had more to do with the inner workings of his own mind than with anything she had done.

Occasionally he seemed to threaten her, but as with an angry child's displeasure, she could defuse the situation with a firm word or by distracting his attention. At times he was inconsolable, so she patiently waited for a better mood to prevail.

Jean was becoming his entire world. If it had been possible, Jean would have stayed home with Manley around the clock. He turned to her for his every need from the moment she opened her eyes in the morning to the moment she dropped off for a fitful few hours of rest at night. He was bitterly resentful when she had to leave for work. The burden was unrelenting. A thousand times she had to tell herself: *It's not Manley. It's the disease.*

He continued his ritual of meeting Jean at work when the weather was decent. Now, of course, he did not drive, so he walked the four miles to Lamb's. Jean would call him when it was time for him to start so that he'd get there at approximately five o'clock, and he would ride home with her in the station wagon. It gave him exercise and something to do. She told him specifically not to come until she had phoned because he had a tendency to start far too early, and then she would either have to keep him occupied at work or stop work to drive him home.

He phoned her frequently at work to hear her voice; this was expressing an infantile need for her reassurance. Once she and her coworkers counted fourteen times that he phoned her at work before noon. As few as five or ten minutes might elapse between calls.

"Hello, Manley," she would say.

"Hi," he would answer. "Talk to you."

"Well, you reached me. Is everything okay?"

"Can I come?" He wanted to start walking to her job now, even though it was still morning, hours too early.

"Not yet, dear. I'll call you when it's time. All right?"

"Yeah." He would be silent, unable to think of anything else to say.

"Well, I have to get back to work," she would tell him.

"All right," he'd respond, satisfied that she was still there. . . until the next phone call.

He began to call and ask where she had gone. It took her awhile to realize that he probably had been dialing wrong numbers. He was losing his ability to make a phone call.

She, in turn, phoned often from Lamb Printing, ever worried that in her absence he would throw himself out an upstairs window or down the stairs. When she returned home at the end of each workday, she experienced a momentary wave of fear when she opened the door, wondering what she'd find. Her worries increased that he would get hit by a car when out walking on his own or would hurt himself at home, either accidentally or intentionally.

During her calls home, she reminded him of things or suggested chores for him to do.

"Why don't you shovel the driveway, Manley?" she might say, or, "There's a new book of word puzzles in the living room on the coffee table."

He still enjoyed working in books of simple word-search puzzles, in which he circled letters in vertical, horizontal, or diagonal lines to form words. When he'd started with these puzzles he could complete an entire book in one day. Now she noted that he had gotten much slower at it; at the end of a day he would only have a single page completed.

As in his healthy past, Manley was never without his comb, handkerchief, and wallet. Even now in his demented state, he always checked his pockets for those items before going outside.

He often misplaced them and would frantically search the house, not satisfied until he found what he was looking for.

He lost his word-search books, too, or a magazine he was perusing. If he put a book or magazine down, he would be unable to find his place in it later, and she would have to help him.

Finding lost objects was more complicated because his verbal powers were minimal, and he would be unable to describe what he was looking for.

"What are you looking for, Manley?"

"You know, you know. . . . I need it."

"What? A tool?"

"Yeah."

"What color is it?"

"Brown." So she and Manley would search everywhere for a brown tool. She made sure that the household was as orderly as possible to minimize these nerve-racking episodes.

A further complication of his diminishing faculties was that he had begun losing his way while walking. He sometimes wandered in circuitous routes and arrived late. Once he mentioned a friend's name and Eagle Street, which was a half mile out of his way to Lamb's. She asked him what he was doing so far off the direct route, and she understood from his answer that he always came that way. Another time he took a wrong turn and ended up in Williamstown, miles past Lamb's. When she got home he wasn't there, but a phone call from the Williamstown police eased her mind. She drove to the police station to pick him up.

Manley's nighttime wandering was a far worse source of trouble. It kept Jean in a constant state of battle readiness and forced her to function on scant hours of sleep, though she would still go to Lamb's the next day because she couldn't afford not to work. She tried everything she could think of, including locking the doors, to keep him inside so she could get her rest, but her efforts usually proved futile if he had his mind set on walking. And she soon discovered that it was a mistake to try to lock him inside. Though he was at a stage now that he couldn't work the locks, he would get so furious that he would almost tear a door off its hinges.

It annoyed Manley when anyone took Jean's attention from him. When she talked to Laurie or to a friend on the phone—or if they were shopping and Jean stopped to talk to an old acquaintance—she had to keep it short or Manley would stomp around in a childish way or try to pull her away. He rarely left her side when they were out together. His delusion that she was carrying on an affair with another man also persisted, despite Jean's efforts to assure him she wasn't. She had learned to accept this lack of trust as a function of the disease.

Jean made sure to keep their daily routine the same. A solid schedule gave him a sense of security and minimized any disorienting surprises. She woke at five o'clock, even though she wasn't due at work till eight, so as to have two and a half hours to prepare Manley for the day. She dressed him in a robe and slippers, and then they ate breakfast. He did better when she ate with him. She saw that he would imitate what she did with the food and utensils. She would fill him with as much food as he would eat because he would forget to feed himself while she was at work.

After breakfast she took her shower, then ran his bath. Baths were easier for him than showers. She stayed in the bathroom to make sure he washed properly. He often resisted washing in the morning, but she coaxed him until he did it. She had to remind him two or three times to brush his teeth and shave. She had to watch him shaving; he had lost the sense of it, and Jean had to get him to go over the parts of his beard he missed. He did it as long as she kept after him.

Next she laid out his clothes in the order that he put things on. Again she had to keep after him as one would a child. He played and dawdled, undoing and redoing his belt or buttons. She was patient, talking to him in a quiet voice so he wouldn't get upset, even if she was getting concerned that she might be late to work. Though his mental capacity was fading, his sensitivity to her was keen; if she lost her temper, he would cry and look forlorn, while she felt her heart would break.

She tied his shoelaces for him. Sometimes he untied them, and she had to tie them again. Lastly she prepared their lunches.

Before leaving she suggested activities for him. "You can play your radio or watch the TV," she would tell him, then leave the television on so he wouldn't have to operate it himself. She would show him a new book of word-search puzzles or a magazine. He still liked to spend time at his workbench in the basement, even if he spent days just sanding a piece of wood. He had started working on a hearth for the wood stove a year before, laying the bricks well enough for a rough, rustic look, but his recent work was wildly uneven and unlevel.

Each month showed proof of his mental erosion. Like a toddler he named things constantly and incessantly asked the same questions: What time is it? What day is it? She wondered if this was an attempt to reassure himself, or if he was reliving the stage in his mental development when he had learned to speak.

"Milk?" he would ask as he picked up his glass of milk.

"Yes, milk," Jean would affirm.

"White?" he said.

"Yes, white."

He picked up a spoon. "Spoon?"

Jean smiled reassuringly. "Spoon, yes. Very good, Manley."

He would smile back and eat with the spoon. Then after an interval he would say it all over again until his attention moved to other objects.

"Milk?" he asked. He was back to his glass of milk.

"Yes. Milk."

"White?"

"Yes."

It was never ending. Jean responded automatically, without thinking, reverting to her days as a young mother caring for her children.

Manley's naming was a background commentary. If they were riding in the car, he would name things he saw.

"Truck?"

"That's right. Truck," she murmured.

He pointed to her yellow blouse. "Yellow?"

"Yes. Yellow."

Pointing to his own shirt, he said, "Blue?"

"That's right, you have a blue shirt on."

Pointing at her blouse again, he said, "Yellow?"

"Yes. Yellow."

"Blue?"

"Blue."

But there were times when he almost perversely seemed to return to a higher level, and he would seem like the Manley of old. At such times Jean experienced sudden hope that his condition could reverse itself.

There was such a day in December when Manley spoke very clearly about what he had done that day.

"I walked . . . town," he said. "Went to post office."

She was stunned. He seemed so happy. His speech was closer to normal again. *He still has ability,* she thought as he continued to relate his activities. *Maybe it's all just stress, and he's snapping out of it.*

"And I had a hot dog. I went Meade Avenue, by old apartment.'' They had lived there after they were married. He also said that he had worked at his workbench, vacuumed, and washed the dishes.

She sat at the kitchen table and listened, light-headed with the happiness of having her beloved soul mate back again. *Maybe he doesn't have Alzheimer's disease! It could be some other illness that's temporary.*

She got up and poured a cup of coffee from a potful that *he* had made. He hadn't done that in a long time, either. He went into the other room to get a magazine he said he'd been reading, and while there, he began to sing. His deep voice filled their house. "You wore a tulip, and I wore a big red rose. . . ."

He knew *all* the lyrics. She hadn't heard him sing in years, let alone remember the lyrics to any songs. Tears of elation filled her eyes. *He's getting better. Everything is going to be all right. Thank you, God.*

But that night it all went away again, and she had to cut up his food and correct the way he held his spoon. This time her tears were for the opposite reason.

CHAPTER 16

Winter
1979

*M*anley had a cousin named Linda Hunt, who lived with her husband and three children in Winthrop, Maine, near Augusta. Jean, Manley, and Steven had visited their home the previous summer on a car trip to see Manley's father. Being fond of Steven, Linda and Jim had talked him into staying with them for a couple of weeks. Steven had enjoyed his time with the family.

Jean and Linda talked by phone periodically, and Linda always asked about Steven. The boy's scholastic performance and general attitude had not improved since he moved in with Bob and Cheryl. When Linda heard about the extent of Steven's problems, she offered to take him into their home. Jean immediately relayed the invitation to Steven, and he jumped at the chance, remembering his fun of the summer before.

When Jean talked it over with Bob MacGowan and Cheryl, Cheryl agreed that a brand-new setting might be beneficial.

Bob opposed the move. He wanted very much to help Steven. It was only December, so Bob felt that he hadn't had enough time to make a difference. Jean assured him that it was not his failure, that the situation was too far advanced already, and that starting fresh in a new school system was worth a try.

In light of Steven's worsening performance in high school, Jean felt she had little choice. She phoned Linda and Jim Hunt and arranged to send Steven to them right after Christmas.

Winthrop, Maine, was smaller in population than North Adams. It lay forty miles from the coast amid densely wooded hilly country with many large lakes.

Jim and Linda's house was in an affluent, rustic part of Winthrop, on a hill outside the center of the village. The first thing

Steven noticed as he got out of the bus after the eight-hour ride was the smell of woodsmoke.

Jim Hunt taught history in the high school, and Linda kept a large house and raised their three children. The eldest, Todd, was Steven's age. His room, which Steven shared, was in the finished basement. He was a little taller than Steven and had a friendly, mild manner. He tended toward intellectual pursuits and despite his large, muscular frame was not an athlete.

Twelve-year-old Jeff was more athletic. Nine-year-old Kim was used to special treatment, being a girl and the youngest. Right away she let Steven know that she would "tell" if anything was done against house rules.

Steven got along particularly well with Jim. Like Steven, he had always been athletically inclined, and they spent much time talking about sports. They also played basketball in the driveway. Even before the warm weather came, Jim was encouraging other boys from the neighborhood to come over and shoot baskets with Steven.

The situation at the high school was very different from what it had been in North Adams. Since Jim was a teacher there, he pre-pared the way for Steven. He was excited that Steven would be pitching for the school baseball team and emphasized that fact as he introduced Steven to the faculty. The school guidance counselor, Timothy Warner, lived across the street from the Hunts and became another ally for the newcomer.

For the first time in years Steven was able to apply himself to his schoolwork and began to perform more like the high achiever he used to be. It was exhilarating to start with a clean slate instead of facing people whose attitudes had been long hardened against him. When his mother phoned weekly to hear how he was doing, he could tell she was relieved and heartened by his progress. It was obvious that moving to Maine had been a wise decision.

In his third week at the new school Steven and a very pretty girl collided in the hallway. She had jet-black hair and lovely dark eyes, a mirror of Steven's coloring. She laughed delightfully and studied him with open curiosity when he apologized for his clumsi-ness. "You're new here, aren't you?"

"Yeah. I'm Steven Tyler."

"I heard you were a friend of Mr. Hunt's."

"I'm staying with him."

"I'm Heidi Webb. Pleased to meet you." She flashed a warm smile, then said, "Gotta run. See you around."

"Bye." Steven watched her walk away down the hall to her class, then turned and dashed to his.

The following day he saw Heidi in the cafeteria and asked if he might sit with her. She was one of the most widely liked girls in the school, and he could understand why. He felt comfortable with her right away and could tell the feeling was mutual.

Heidi didn't have a boyfriend, so he asked her to go with him to a home basketball game. She accepted.

After their date, they talked for hours over ice cream in a local restaurant.

"I can see you love basketball," Heidi said. "Did you play at your old high school?"

"Some, yes. But mostly I played at the Y."

"Why not at school?"

"I guess I didn't like my coaches."

"Why not?"

He thought for a moment about how to answer her without explaining his life story. "Things were different there," he said finally. "We didn't get along too well."

"Why not? You're a nice person."

"They didn't think so."

She looked quizzically at him then, trying to discern some dark, hidden danger about him. Finally she satisfied herself there was none. "Why don't you play here?"

"I'm not eligible because I moved here after the season started. But I'll try out for baseball in the spring."

They talked seriously, watching each other intently, learning about one another bit by bit. Steven found himself wanting to share some of his deepest thoughts with her. Her questions seemed based in real interest rather than idle curiosity.

Walking Heidi home, Steven realized he was happy. Being at her side, strolling along the quiet avenue, he felt protective and chivalrous, as he imagined an adult might feel.

At her front door he took her hand and squeezed it. The gesture had more warmth than a normal handshake, and they gravitated closer. He hadn't hoped to kiss her, but she seemed to invite it. He did, simply, on the lips, then took a step back. All he could think to say was, "It was a fun night."

She smiled happily. "Wasn't it? See you Monday." She went inside.

Steven enjoyed the four-mile walk to the Hunts' house, replaying the entire evening in his mind and grinning. It was hard for him to believe that he could suddenly feel so happy in this strange little town so far from his real home, but he undeniably did.

In the peaceful weeks that followed, Steven found himself rediscovering aspects of his personality that he had thought were gone forever. Once again his teachers, coaches, and other adults were friends and helpers. When he participated in the normal classroom give-and-take, it was as if the cooperative, friendly boy he used to be was reemerging after a long hibernation.

He found that he was eager to please again. His cynicism vanished. Sometimes he thought about his father, but usually his thoughts of home revolved around his mother. He hoped she was all right by herself.

The normality of the Hunt household was calming for him. Jim liked him and treated him well. Steven had forgotten what petty sibling rivalries were like. The Hunts' worst squabbles were tame in comparison to what he'd lived through with his parents.

An added bonus was Mr. Warner across the street. The guidance counselor took a special interest in Steven. The boy had to shake his head at the crazy contrasts in his life. Suddenly he was liked again by adults and kids.

For the first few weeks in the new house the old feelings would return at moments. But they were fading away. He couldn't remember when he'd been happier. He felt sorry for his parents but couldn't help enjoying his new home and his beautiful girlfriend. Heidi made him feel strong and whole, happy to be alive.

He enjoyed being normal again and put real effort into his schoolwork. He rediscovered the satisfaction of being a bright student instead of an antisocial misanthrope.

Even gym class was different for him. He had gotten so accustomed to being an outsider that he had to relearn what it was like to be a willing volunteer for athletic activities instead of a grudging participant with coaches who "had it in for him." Now he was accepted as part of the group, another good player. He had no need to walk around with a chip on his shoulder. It felt terrific.

With this distance from his hometown, Steven realized how heavily his burdens had been weighing on him. No students called him geek or a troublemaker. *Maybe I'm not such a bad person after all,* he mused. It made sense that he should find peace here, twenty miles from Augusta, where his father was born.

After Christmas Jean took two of the three weeks she was allotted for vacation time. She had thought it would be nice for Manley to have her at home during the holidays. During the two weeks she was able to watch her husband's behavior around the clock, she found that his abilities had deteriorated more than she thought.

He did almost no activity on his own. If she sat in the kitchen, he did, too. If she got up and walked into the den or upstairs or outside, he followed. If she got up from the kitchen table and went to the cabinets across the room, when she turned around he was right behind her, almost touching her. She did her best to include him. When she did the laundry, she let him load items into the washing machine.

More often than not he needed help using eating utensils. He would try to use a knife when he really needed a fork or spoon, or he'd hold a spoon or fork the wrong way around and try to balance food on the handle. His muscles were familiar with the required movements, but his confused brain was less able to sort out the proper procedure for a given need. Manley's cutting meat was out of the question. If she cut it up for him, however, he could get it to his mouth with a fork or spoon or, increasingly, with his fingers.

He needed constant monitoring. He sprinkled sugar on soup or salt on cereal. If he wanted something, he would point and say, "I want. It, want it."

She was with Manley twenty-four hours a day, and the work was never ending. There were few moments when he wasn't at her side. It got on her nerves, but as at every other stage in his decline, she adapted as best she could. Her only respite was when she could get him to sleep or interest him in television for a while. It was exhausting.

After just a few days at home Jean was forced to admit that her husband could not be left alone and unattended. It wasn't fair to him, and it was potentially dangerous.

It was 1980; almost nine years had elapsed since Manley's abrupt resignation from the educational system had begun the dismantling of their lives. She thought long and hard about her options. She had to work; their savings were gone, and expenses continued. It was clear that Manley would have to be cared for by someone while Jean was at her workplace. She began inquiring about getting help.

Dr. Ellis suggested local organizations and services. Jean called the Visiting Nurses Association, Elder Services, and the Department of Mental Health. The VNA would charge more for their assistance than the five dollars an hour Jean earned at Lamb's. Representatives of Elder Services and the Department of Mental Health interviewed Manley and concluded that he was too impaired to be admitted to their facilities. They could not provide the one-on-one supervision his condition required.

Instead, Jean was offered counseling for herself. She attended a few group meetings and talked to professionals about her problem, but it was soon clear that she knew more about caregiving than anyone to whom she spoke. No one she talked to had heard of Alzheimer's disease. When Jean described Manley's behavior, people thought she was describing schizophrenia or another mental illness, and she spent frustrating hours trying to educate them on the differences.

Having given up on community-service organizations, Jean placed a small advertisement in the local newspaper, asking for someone to care for her husband while she worked. She got some responses, primarily from retired women, but once they met Manley and learned the extent of his problem, the applicants declined the position. They seemed intimidated that mental problems were involved.

Jean, at a loss, sought the advice of her relatives, including Manley's aunt Charlotte.

Charlotte Exford was a younger sister of Manley's mother. Charlotte, her husband, and their daughters, Sandra and Diane, had lived right next door for much of Manley's childhood. Charlotte's husband had died years before, but she still lived in their house with her daughter Diane, who had cerebral palsy but functioned well despite mild mental retardation. Charlotte worked afternoons for Elder Services, delivering Meals-on-Wheels, a food service for the elderly.

Charlotte offered to supervise Manley every morning, before she went to her afternoon job. Having known Manley nearly all his life and having had extensive experience with the retarded, she was well qualified to help. Also, Charlotte expected no pay, knowing that Jean's financial status was precarious.

Jean couldn't believe her good fortune and thanked God for Charlotte's selfless generosity. It was decided that Jean would work half a day if her employers were agreeable. She talked to Bob Lamb, the elder brother managing Lamb Printing. He was glad to keep her on part-time and magnanimously offered to continue providing full health-insurance coverage.

Charlotte came every morning. She drove Jean to work and

took Manley to her own house for half a day, then picked Jean up at noontime and dropped Manley and her off at home again.

Now reduced to earning half a day's pay, Jean kept creditors at bay by paying small amounts toward her bills while the family's debts continued to grow.

CHAPTER 17

Spring
1980

*J*ean was very appreciative of Charlotte's assistance, but caring for Manley the rest of the time became more trying. The hours she spent at work were a welcome break from her ceaseless vigilance at home.

Since Jean was with her husband for more hours than before, she would take him on long walks all over Clarksburg and North Adams when weather permitted. She knew he enjoyed it, and he seemed less inclined to wander at night if he had had a four- or five-mile walk during the day.

Because of her constant concern for Manley, Steven's improvement was a tremendous relief for Jean. She was intrigued that he had a steady girlfriend; until now his relationships with girls had been strictly temporary. And on 28 January 1980 Laurie DelNegro gave birth to a healthy baby girl, whom she and Art named Katie Jean. *Thank God a few things are going right for a change,* she thought.

In February she decided to take a week off work and take Manley to visit Steven in Winthrop.

The winter landscape raced past the window as the bus barreled along through the New England countryside. It had been hours since the vehicle left Boston, and it would be another hour or more until it reached North Adams on the return trip from Winthrop, Maine, where Jean and Manley had been for five days.

Manley had been happy enough in the company of his cousins Jim and Linda and their children. His contribution to the conversations was limited to occasional short phrases, leaving the listener to guess the rest of what he had meant to say. Manley understood few subtleties of the conversation, but when there was laughter, he would join in. He had remained on the periphery of activity, doing his customary pacing in the unfamiliar house. At meals he often got up for no reason and walked away from the table with his meal only half-eaten. They would hear him walking back and forth in the next room.

From the first day Manley had worried obsessively about the bathroom. He would walk to it, look inside, then walk away again. Five minutes later he repeated the behavior. Jean realized that he was reassuring himself where the bathroom was located, since his short-term memory was so poor now. The Hunts had been very understanding and patient about all his anomalies.

During the visit Steven had taken his mother aside and confided that something was wrong in Jim and Linda's relationship. Todd and he had frequently heard the married couple arguing heatedly. Jean had explained to Steven that it was normal for husbands and wives to argue, although he hadn't witnessed much of that in her once-happy marriage.

The stay in Winthrop had been passably pleasant, but the bus rides had been hellish. Manley had disliked sitting motionless for so long in the narrow seat. The trip from North Adams to Boston had lasted three and a half hours, with a half-hour stopover, then another three hours to Winthrop.

Manley's obsession with bathrooms took on nightmarish proportions while traveling. Every ten minutes he would walk up and back in the narrow bus aisle, nervously reminding himself where the tiny facility was located. When he went into the bathroom, he sometimes stayed far longer than necessary, and Jean had to talk to him through the door while everyone around her listened. A couple of times she enlisted the assistance of other men if Manley couldn't figure out how things operated in the unfamiliar cubicle.

The men's room tribulations were not limited to the bus ride. While waiting at the Boston bus terminal Jean had shown him to the bathroom, and he'd gone inside alone. As the minutes ticked by she had grown increasingly nervous, but she couldn't go into a men's room to find him. Finally she had sought the help of a kindly looking passerby. The gentleman graciously brought Manley out, saying that he'd been wandering around the large room, evidently unable to find the exit.

Jean sighed now with exhaustion as Manley fidgeted beside her, glancing out the window, then looking around at the other passengers, then out the window again. He shifted his feet and tapped his fingers on the armrest. Then he started to stand. If she'd had any idea how difficult it would be traveling with her husband, she would never have made the trip.

"Where are you going, hon?" Jean asked, barely containing her exasperation.

"Bathroom," he said.

"But you just went twenty minutes ago."

He looked around, motioning impatiently with his hand. "Bathroom!"

"Manley, please wait awhile. It's not fair to the other passengers to be using it constantly like this. Look out the window, dear. Please."

But he was single-minded and willful. He pushed past her into the narrow aisle, and she could do nothing to stop him. He walked the few feet to the lavatory, oblivious to the curious or annoyed expressions of the other travelers. She heard the door of the cubicle close and felt thankful that it wasn't already occupied.

The shortness of Manley's attention span was much more obvious to Jean away from home. In the familiar surroundings of home, he didn't have the difficulty that he was experiencing now.

When Manley had been gone long enough, Jean rose from her seat and made her way to the lavatory as the bus rocked over the highway. A man was waiting outside the cubicle. Jean went to the door and knocked.

"Manley?" She heard a mumbled answer from within. "Come on out now, dear. Someone is waiting." She smiled an apology to the man. When she heard nothing from within, she knocked again. "Do you need help, Manley?"

"Yes," came the muffled response. She debated whether she should go in, but the man beside her offered to help. "I'll go in and help him, if you want. I've had some experience with the retarded."

"Thank you," Jean answered. She was getting used to people's assumption that Manley was retarded. The doorknob was not locked. As the man entered, Jean could see that Manley was standing over the tiny sink, staring into it. The door closed, and she heard the man speaking quietly. Manley came out a minute later, and she led him back to their seat. One thing she knew for a certainty: She was never going on a bus trip with him again.

Aunt Charlotte found that caring for Manley did not pose any difficulty. He obeyed her requests and was well-behaved. He reminded Charlotte so much of the way he had been as a boy, always the little gentleman. It saddened her that Manley had come to this turn in life.

When he had briefly taught a woodworking class to retarded adults, his cousin Diane worked in the kitchen in the same facility. She had told her mother that Manley would sometimes get very angry and yell at his students. This hadn't sounded like the Manley Charlotte knew—the Manley who used to teach Sunday school and take children on marvelous field trips to Boston.

Not so many months before Manley had visited her on occasion, during his long daytime walks. He hadn't seemed so bad. It pained her that people in the community so misunderstood his problem. For example, an acquaintance had called Charlotte to ask directions, and she had suggested that the man call Manley because he knew how to get there and was much better than she was at giving directions. The acquaintance had stunned her when he'd said, "Oh, no. I'm not going to call Manley. He's nothing but an old drunk." Charlotte was learning about the strange things this illness did to the mind. Although Jean had told her about Manley's delusions, Charlotte was shocked by them.

Though Jean tried to prepare her, Charlotte had not expected Manley's condition to be so severe. She brought her nephew on errands around town and for walks and picnics. If she had to run into a store for a few minutes, he would wait obediently in the car. She kept his attention occupied and his energies engaged. He enjoyed their outings. One of his favorite places to go was the Apothecary Hall, a drugstore in downtown North Adams that made mocha sundaes, one of Manley's favorites.

Charlotte saw that her nephew had very little short-term memory, but he remembered things that transpired far back in time. Around town he encountered people he had known all his life. Although it was obvious that he wasn't the Manley of old, he recognized most of his longtime acquaintances during chance meetings and returned their greetings with a smile.

At Charlotte's home, however, Manley was less content. He would sit and stare for a long time, and he cried a great deal, quietly, to himself. Sometimes he would go into her bedroom for a nap, and Charlotte would look in on him and find tears streaming down his face. Occasionally she would hear him mumbling unhappily, and every now and then she heard the word *boyfriend*. She would console him and assure him things would be all right, and sometimes that lifted his dark mood.

162

Often Manley's distress was so bad Charlotte had to call Jean at work and ask her advice. Jean would talk to Manley, reassuring him that she loved him, that she was at work and would see him later. That would usually appease him. But there were times when he wasn't so easily mollified, and Jean had to leave work for the day to be with him.

Charlotte couldn't imagine what kind of nightmare Jean had been living all this time, nor how she could stand it. She had been such a good wife and mother—it just wasn't fair.

In the past Jean had joked to Angie about taking things one month at a time. Now it seemed she could barely think a week in advance. Jean sometimes wondered at the life she now led. When she wasn't overwhelmed with sadness and could view herself with some objectivity, it boggled her mind that all this had happened. She was a patient woman and had been raised to be hardworking and optimistic; but an anger was growing in her. If Manley had to die—and Dr. Ellis told her from the first that death was unavoidable—better that he would have died of a heart attack, cancer . . . anything was better than watching someone die the slowest death imaginable. Alzheimer's was unending, insidious torture. Hour by hour, day by day, a little more of the self vanished.

What can possibly happen next? she wondered. Whenever she thought it couldn't get any worse, it did.

Jean no longer got proper rest. For a time after Manley was diagnosed, he slept normal hours. But now there was no set pattern, so Jean never went to bed with the intention of sleeping. Instead she would lie in bed, reading and listening, and might doze off for a few hours if she was lucky. Her subconscious remained on alert for sounds of movement, and she awoke at all hours of the night to check on Manley as he paced the house, hit the walls, and moved objects.

Although it made Manley panicky to have doors locked, she risked locking the two outer doors at night. This way, if she did fall asleep and he tried to leave the house, she would be awakened by the ruckus of his being locked in. Then she would either talk him out of leaving or have to let him out and, of course, follow him. Thankfully, his nighttime treks had tapered off considerably . . . perhaps because Jean did so much walking with him during the day.

It took hours every day now for just the most basic life-sustaining activities. Jean had to squeeze the toothpaste on the toothbrush, hand it to Manley, and keep after him until his teeth were cleaned.

He would not bathe himself anymore. Jean had to get into the shower with her husband and wash him. Sometimes he resisted bathing, so she gave up for the moment and tried again later. She always managed to get him washed. Months later it dawned on her why he disliked bathing: He had come to associate it with being separated from her. When she made him take a shower, he knew that she would soon be leaving for work. After Jean realized this, she began bathing him in the evening and found him far less resistant.

Dressing was getting more difficult. After ten minutes he might remove most of his clothes or add more garments. Many times she had to laugh when he put jockey shorts on over his trousers. She simplified his clothes to make it easier for him, giving him cardigans instead of pullover sweaters, loafers instead of shoes that had laces. She also dispensed with his belt, since it was a source of frustration.

Thankfully, he never wet the bed. He worked hard at avoiding accidents and often went into the hall to assure himself that the bathroom was still there. Unfortunately, he was occasionally incontinent. He would be on the way to the bathroom to urinate, but his mind, so easily distracted, forgot, and he wet his pants. He would look terribly sad, knowing he had done something shameful. "I'm bad," he'd say. "Bad."

Jean would feel profoundly sorry for him in those moments. It was necessary, of course, to undress him and bathe him and dress him yet again—all with smiles and gentleness, trying not to show displeasure or anger. Jean always apologized to *him* for the humiliation.

CHAPTER 18

Early 1980

*L*aurie smiled as she watched Manley wheeling baby Kate around the living room in her stroller. He looked so happy with his granddaughter. Manley was staying the night to give Jean a rare evening out with friends. Laurie, having seen the signs of tremendous strain on her mother, had made all the arrangements.

"Okay, you two, time for dinner." She picked her daughter up. "C'mon, Dad. You must be hungry."

"Hungry, hungry," he said, then followed her dutifully. They sat at the dining room table. Art was waiting for them.

Laurie watched Manley as he took a seat next to Kate's high chair. She remembered the days when her father was strong and wise. All her life she had been his little girl. Now she was like a mother to him.

"Chow time," Art said genially. "Smells great, Laur. Special just for you, Manley."

Manley looked at Art, then back at the plates heaped with steaming food.

As they ate, Laurie watched her father. He looked so robust, it made her feel good. He'd bounce back; she was sure of it. He had to—he was still so young and healthy.

After dinner, Art found a basketball game on television while Laurie put Kate to sleep. Manley was absorbed in the game, and when Art made comments about the Celtics, Manley didn't respond. Art guessed his father-in-law was attracted merely by the movement.

Art was worried about his wife. Laurie seemed unable to accept the obvious regarding her father. She still got angry if he remarked that Manley was worse or that Manley might have to be institutionalized. Art could understand her reluctance to face reality, but it wasn't healthy to avoid the facts, either. Denial wouldn't change anything, and it might be worse for her in the long run. Jean, Laurie, and Steven were all fighting the inevitable in their own way, refusing to give in. But one of these days, Art knew, they'd have little choice.

When it was time for bed, Laurie walked Manley upstairs to the guest room.

"This is your bed, Dad." She turned down the quilt and fluffed the pillows. "Want to brush your teeth now?" He followed her out to the bathroom, and she put toothpaste on the brush for him. He put the toothbrush in his mouth but didn't do much with it.

"Go ahead, Dad. Brush. Want to keep those teeth clean." She took his hand and moved it up and down, showing him how. Then she helped him rinse his mouth, making a mess over the sink.

Back in the bedroom she said, "Here are the pajamas Mom brought for you. Can you do it?"

He stared at her.

"It's time to get undressed now, Dad. Put on your pajamas." She sighed as she realized he needed assistance getting undressed. "I'll help you."

When he was in his pajamas, she kissed him.

He smiled but just stood in the middle of the room.

"You have to go to bed now, Dad."

The look on his face changed to perplexity. Then a measure of comprehension came into his eyes, and with it came wrenching distress, as if part of him perceived the humiliation of this moment.

"Good night, Dad. Sleep tight." She kissed him again, then fled the room, closing the door behind her.

In her own bedroom she sat down and cried quietly. Art came in, and she pulled herself together before he noticed her misery. She took out a book and feigned reading. Then when they turned out the lights, she listened to the silence. When Art's breathing lengthened and deepened, she slipped out of bed and left the room. She knew she would not be sleeping for some time. Her father might get up and go looking for the bathroom.

The door to his room was at the head of the stairs, and she worried that he might fall down the steps. She went into the living room and waited, all her senses alert so she could help her father when he needed it.

Part of her admitted that her father was much worse than he had been only months before, but part of her believed he might still recover his mental capacities and prove the know-it-all doctors wrong. Thinking the best might make everything all right.

Hours later she went up to bed, but she kept her door open so she could see her father's room. She finally got a little sleep as the faintest gray light became visible outside.

In late March Jean received unsettling news from Linda Hunt in Winthrop, Maine. She and her husband, Jim, were separating. This meant that Steven would have to come home.

Oh, no, Jean thought, *this can't be happening to Steven.* She sat in her kitchen, dumbfounded. *Can't anything go right for that poor boy?*

Two days later Jean received a call from Timothy Warner, the high-school guidance counselor who lived on the same street as the Hunts.

"Steven is a great kid, Mrs. Tyler. He has been through an awful lot for someone so young, though, and I'm afraid he'll feel responsible for Jim and Linda's breakup. Wherever he goes, things seem to fall apart. He's got enough on his mind without guilt about that."

A few weeks later Steven boarded a bus and left Winthrop, Maine, and Heidi Webb behind him. She had cried when he said good-bye to her. Heidi had given him a feeling of completeness. Now he felt numb and disoriented. He knew he would miss her, but he accepted the separation with the same detachment he'd had for all the other bad things that life had thrown his way. He hadn't even had the opportunity to play baseball, as he'd been looking forward to all winter.

As the bus brought him closer to his old life, he thought about the past few months. He felt older and wiser, but an unsettling nervousness grew inside him as the miles sped by.

When the bus rolled into North Adams, his life of normalcy in Winthrop seemed far away and dreamlike. As he saw the familiar streets and buildings, the old Steven Tyler began to reemerge: the rebel . . . the brooding, unreachable cynic.

"Steven, you've got to go back to school," Jean told him a few days after his arrival.

"I don't want to."

"You have no choice. You've got to get your education."

Jean felt the same way about the school that Steven did. She didn't want him to go back there, either, but she saw no alternative. "Please, Steven. Maybe it'll be better now. You don't have much more time left—next year you graduate."

He finally went back to school. He began to connect again with old friends and enemies. He used his mother's car legally now, but in typical youthful fashion he was brutal with it, untroubled that he was contributing to the mechanical troubles that kept it in the repair shop.

Steven tried to be available during the afternoons so that his mother could do errands while he supervised his father. Manley, Steven noticed, didn't seem to resent him as much. Seeing how bad his father's condition was, Steven felt sad and impotent.

Not long after his return from Maine, Steven made a new friend, Mike Fierro, at Drury High School. Mike, a year younger than Steven, lived ten miles north in Stamford, Vermont.

Mike's father, Dave, was an athletically built, earthy man of vitality and humor. He was a disc jockey for a North Adams radio station that played rock and roll. When Mike brought Steven home with him, Dave took an immediate dislike to his son's new friend. Steven had gotten into the habit of speaking flippantly, what Dave called "shooting off his mouth."

Dave was not one to disguise his feelings, and Steven got the message. The next time he went home with Mike, Steven treated Dave Fierro with respect and deference. This time Dave was impressed by Steven's quick mind and sincerity.

From that day on, Steven became very close with the whole Fierro family. To Dave it was like having another son, which he didn't mind at all. He called Steven "Tippy," after the historic political slogan: Tippecanoe and Tyler Too.

Mike also spent time at the Tyler household. Steven would make light of Manley's disease. He got into the habit of making fun of his father, although he didn't do it in his mother's presence. One of Steven's antics was to say obscene things and curse in front of his father, and when Manley didn't respond, he and Mike would laugh.

Jean liked it when Steven and Mike stayed overnight on old couches in the basement family room. She knew Steven couldn't get into trouble while he stayed at home. He was hardly ever at home otherwise.

Jean liked Mike and was thankful that Steven had a family to be with, but she worried about what he did the rest of the time. Some of the boys with whom Steven was friendly made her nervous. She had heard the names of many of them in connection with wildness and trouble with the law. And sadly, all contact between Steven and Heidi Webb ended when he left Maine.

CHAPTER 19

Summer 1981

One summer day Manley watched as Steven cut the lawn. It must have reminded him that he wasn't upholding his own responsibilities because he came outside and took the power mower away. As Steven watched, Manley mowed in a straight line to the road, then he stopped and stood there, unable to continue.

Later, Steven described the experience to his mother. "He didn't even know enough to turn the mower around to do the next row."

"I know," she said. "I've seen him do that before. I just go and turn him around, and he does another row."

Dr. Jay Ellis was becoming as much of a family friend as a consulting neurologist. He had ceased to treat Manley Tyler. Now he was treating Jean and her children. In the summer of 1981 he again suggested that she seek long-term professional care for Manley.

"You should do it fairly soon," he advised her. "With your financial pressures, problems with Steven, lack of sleep, and everything else you are suffering, it is madness to allow the situation to continue."

She nodded at his irrefutable logic, but this was her husband he was talking about. She was not about to shift her burden to some anonymous staff of orderlies and nurses until she had absolutely no choice. Her presence comforted Manley; her absence might have the opposite effect.

Jay read the resistance in her expression. He did not want to see her destroyed along with her husband. "Jean, listen to me: The slowness of the disease often gives people false hope, as if the condition has stabilized. But I've never heard of a case of remission for Alzheimer's. I don't want you to suffer unnecessarily. Besides, Manley is less and less aware of what's going on. You can visit him every day if you wish—spend all the time you want. Before long it won't matter to him, and it will be much easier on you and Steven."

"I appreciate your concern, Jay. I'll do what's necessary when the time comes. I'm sure I'll know it when it happens."

Jay wasn't so sure, but he admired Jean's tenacious loyalty to the man she loved.

She gazed into the face of her handsome husband as they danced dreamily across the large balcony. His eyes sparkled with wisdom and good humor.

"I'm glad you're back," Jean said happily. "I missed you. God, how I missed you."

Manley laughed deeply, heartily. "You know I'll never leave you."

Then he drew her close, putting his lips on hers in the gentlest kiss she could remember. There was so much she wanted to tell him and even more she wanted to ask. Did you know what's been going on? What was it like? How did you feel? Did you know that I never stopped loving you? Is it over now?

His lips left hers, and he answered her thoughts with a loving smile that filled her with contentment. "I'll always love you," he promised.

"And I you."

A shooting star streaked across the night sky, and tears of joy rolled down her face. She held on to him tightly and breathed into his ear, "I'm so glad you're back, Manley. . . ."

Movement in the room awakened her from her dream. Peace was replaced by dread as she watched Manley disappear through the doorway. She closed her eyes and listened as he searched the hallway of the rented cottage, looking for the bathroom.

How long had she slept? By her clock on the nightstand it was three in the morning. She had gotten over three hours of sleep. *Not bad, but not enough.*

She sat up and slipped her feet into her tennis shoes. She had come to hate this bedroom and the whole cottage. She and Manley were vacationing on the coast of Maine. Aunt Charlotte and Cousin Diane were asleep across the hall . . . if Manley hadn't awakened them.

They had been there for eleven days . . . the worst eleven days

Jean had ever experienced. Manley had been unable to adjust to the new surroundings and had not given them an hour's peace.

It had seemed like a good idea back in Clarksburg. Charlotte was taking a vacation with Diane and suggested that Manley might like to see the seashore of Maine, which he'd loved all his life. Jean was willing to try anything that might give her husband some pleasure, that might stir some pleasant memories. But she couldn't have made a worse decision.

She took her robe from a chair and went into the hall. Manley was shuffling along, touching the wall with his hand. She took his arm.

"This way, dear," she whispered, and led him in the opposite direction, into the bathroom. She closed the door and waited for him outside.

It amazed her that he couldn't remember where the bathroom was from hour to hour even though they'd been here for so many days and never turned the bathroom light off. Such a total lack of memory was hard to comprehend.

In a week and a half Jean had learned a difficult lesson: A person with Alzheimer's disease suffered doubly in unfamiliar surroundings. Looking back, she knew she should have realized that from their terrible bus trip to and from Winthrop. On the other hand, he hadn't been too bad at the Hunt household for four days, so she assumed he would eventually get acclimated at the cottage. She could have kicked herself for her foolishness. The days had been hellish.

Since their arrival, Manley had been in a state of unremitting misery, roaming wildly around the cottage, bewildered by everything. He went outside to walk in the sand and pebbles, but the views and fresh sea air had no beneficial effect. With the loss of brain function, he evidently lost the ability to enjoy even so elementary a pleasure as the seashore. He was horribly upset that he didn't know where he was.

To make matters worse, Manley developed a terrible toothache almost immediately. When Jean and Charlotte asked him what was wrong, he could only groan and point to his jaw.

"Hurts," he moaned, bursting into tears. "Hurts."

In addition he seemed to have pain in his abdomen. He hardly slept at all, keeping a raw edge to Jean's nerves.

They located a local dentist who thoroughly examined Manley but found nothing wrong. He was going to prescribe some painkillers, but when Jean told him about the medication she had brought for Manley, the dentist thought better of it and suggested that the cause was psychosomatic.

That may be true, Jean had thought, *but the pain is real to Manley.*

They brought Manley to the dentist four times, but no physical cause could be found. Aspirin did nothing, nor did the tranquilizers Jean had packed for the trip. Manley would wake in the middle of the night and pace and moan pitifully, hitting walls and doors with his hands.

One night he moaned so piteously while holding his stomach that Charlotte and she had taken him to the nearest emergency room. A doctor had examined him, but he couldn't find anything wrong with Manley, either.

Jean couldn't wait to get home. The cottage kitchen was equipped with only the bare essentials, so making him the countless snacks and meals that helped consume his time was difficult. There was no television or radio.

When she brought him to an inlet pool to swim, she thought he'd remember his love of swimming. But he put his foot into the water once and drew it back with distaste, and that was as wet as he got.

She heard Manley moaning now behind the bathroom door, so she went inside. He was sitting on the edge of the tub, holding his face and rocking. She flushed the toilet for him and helped him up. Though she tried to be quiet, their passage down the hall was noisy. She got him into the bedroom and told him to lie down, but it was no good; he would be up for hours. His expression was contorted, and he writhed angrily and turned his head this way and that.

"Hurts! Hurts!" he cried loudly.

She sat beside him and tried to comfort him, massaging his shoulders and neck, hopeful of getting him more relaxed. But he sat up a moment later and moaned again. She asked him to lie down, but he got angry.

"No!"

He got up and began walking the floor. She decided to give him a snack; maybe that would settle him. She had gotten used to the routine: Try this, try that, keep him occupied as much as possible, and the time would pass . . . eventually.

She led him into the kitchen, brought him cheese and crackers at the table, then poured him a glass of milk. A few minutes later Manley's aunt joined them in the kitchen.

"Up again, I see." Charlotte said sleepily. "Is he still in pain?"

173

"Yes. Sorry, Charlotte. I tried to keep him quiet—"

"I know, dear. Nothing you can do about it. That's the way things are. Some vacation, huh?"

Jean snorted. "A barrel of laughs. Sun and fun."

Charlotte filled a kettle with water. "Well, how could we have known? We have two more days. Do you want to go back sooner?"

Jean did, but she didn't want to deprive Charlotte and Diane of their vacation.

"No," she said. "I can stick it out if you can."

"It's hardest on you, Jean." The water in the kettle started to boil. "Want a cup of tea?"

"Sure. Thanks, Charlotte. Well, where do you want to go next year? A cruise, maybe?"

They drove home two days later. Once Manley was back in North Adams, his pains vanished. Jean did not want to take chances, however, and sought Dr. Everett's advice. He arranged for Manley to be admitted to the North Adams Regional Hospital for testing.

Dr. Everett had a secondary reason for admitting Manley: He wanted to give Jean a few days of much needed rest. He had observed that the course of Manley's decline was taking a heavy toll on her, and despite his warnings, she seemed to ignore her own needs.

Now, for the first time in weeks, Jean had a few days to sleep undisturbed. She talked to Angie Potter on the phone during the interlude and was able to laugh about the trip to the seashore.

"I can laugh now, but a few days ago I was ready to commit suicide or murder—it didn't matter which one."

"How long is this going to continue, Jean?" Angie asked. "How much more can you take?"

Jean made light of it. "Oh, it's not so bad. I'll be better now that we're home again. Manley will be back in the surroundings he's used to, and, I hope, he'll be back to normal." She chuckled with black humor and repeated the word ironically. "*Normal.*"

Angie said, "One person's normal is another's off-the-wall. It's all a matter of perspective, I guess."

Jean shook her head. "How could I have expected Manley to enjoy a trip like that? Sometimes I think I'm brain damaged myself."

Angie quipped, "What do you expect of two people born in the year of the chicken?"

Jean had a good laugh for the first time in weeks. A local Chi-

174

nese restaurant had place mats that gave designations from Chinese culture corresponding to the year of one's birth. She and Angie had both been born in the year of the chicken.

During Manley's hospital stay numerous tests were performed. Nothing out of the ordinary was found. He seemed to be in excellent health, physically.

Manley's five-day stay caused disruptions, however. The nurses complained to Jean that he wandered around the hospital, bothering other patients. He had caused no end of trouble and was uncooperative to the point of violence. The more forceful they became, the more stubborn and hostile he reacted.

Jean had learned that most professionals, be they doctors or nurses, knew almost nothing about the behavior and needs of an Alzheimer's patient. The staff at North Adams Regional Hospital was no exception.

She tried her best to explain about his illness, but the staff didn't know what she was talking about. They had no training for such a contingency. They were thankful that Jean spent so much time at the hospital, since she was the only person to whom Manley would respond.

She stayed for hours, sitting with him, walking in the halls, and helping him eat. He seemed to have trouble eating, which puzzled Jean. His appetite was one thing that wasn't affected by the illness. One day, after a typical hospital dinner had been set in front of him, he stared at the tray with its multiple plates and containers, then flung the entire array across the room.

Jean cleaned it up and brought a still-intact container of pudding back to his bed. To her surprise he started to eat it with gusto. She obtained another dinner for him, but this time she gave him only one item at a time. He ate with his normal appetite. She realized that he had been confused by the many different types of food. His mind rebelled at having to make choices, but having one food in front of him at a time made it possible for him to eat.

While she was at the hospital, Jean asked a staff social worker for information on institutions where Alzheimer's patients could be placed. The woman didn't know a thing about Alzheimer's but suggested that they look into nursing homes and state or federally funded hospitals. She told Jean that placement often required a long processing time and suggested Jean begin applying now. She obtained various forms to be filled out to start the procedure.

CHAPTER 20

Summer
1981

After his hospitalization Manley's level of functioning dropped significantly. For the first time Jean noticed a slight shuffle in his walk. She was also aware of a sagging and a twitching on one side of his face.

Jean had to do everything for him now. She washed him, shaved him, even brushed his teeth, which was no easy feat, since she was shorter than he and had to stand behind him to do it.

He needed help in every stage of dressing but was still adept at removing his clothes, which he did often.

She fed him one kind of food at a time. Much of it could be handled with his fingers. The use of fork, knife, and spoon confounded him now.

Manley's bad moods began to express themselves in more frightening episodes. He was physically aggressive toward Jean. She might be standing at the stove or sink, and he would come over and hit her on the shoulder with his hand—not hard enough to cause any real pain but in a childlike display of petulant displeasure. Then one day he pushed her hard, sending her against a cabinet with a crash.

Sudden eruptions of anger occurred with more and more frequency. She would get out of his way then say, "Don't be like that, Manley. You know I'm doing the best I can for you."

But he had his tender moments, too, when he would feel sorry and repentant, or when he seemed suddenly to remember who he was. Then he would touch her gently and say, "Good. Good."

She knew what he meant, even though he couldn't say the words: It was the same as when he used to tell her that she was so good to him, even *too* good for him, when he was feeling sorry for himself.

Because Manley was abusive, Jean became more wary, looking around for him, wondering what he'd do next. She slept even less than she had before, drifting off then snapping awake.

One night she had drifted off to sleep with the television on and with Manley beside her. She was awakened as she suddenly hit the floor beside the bed.

She rubbed her side and looked at him. "Why did you knock me out of bed, Manley?"

He just stared at her with a look mean enough to give her chills. She left the room and lay down on the couch in the living room but barely slept. A week later she again woke up as she hit the floor next to the bed.

There were times when she came close to losing her steadfast affection for Manley. One night after a week of sleepless nights she felt such rage that she went into the bathroom, stuffed a towel into her mouth, and screamed.

His obsession with locating the bathroom now occurred at home as well as elsewhere. He repeatedly walked to the central hall-way, stopped in front of the bathroom door, went away, then came back. On certain days he seemed to do nothing else. Jean occasion-ally found him pacing in front of the door with increasing urgency, needing to use the bathroom yet not seeming to know to go in.

Always vigilant, she began to take him to the bathroom often during the day, wanting to prevent incidents of incontinence. This was for Manley as well as for herself; he felt humiliated when he uri-nated on himself. Because of her efforts, accidents seldom hap-pened.

At this point he rarely put more than two words together. The words might or might not make sense. But Jean usually knew what he was trying to say from his body language or where he was look-ing. The context also helped: what time of day or night it was, what was happening right at the moment.

One morning after a typical night of fitful sleep, Jean walked into the kitchen and greeted Manley, who was wearing his brown velour robe. As she went by to the sink, she noticed a glint of metal from inside his flared sleeve.

Suddenly wary, she turned to him and smiled. Her own non-chalance amazed her. "What've you got there, Manley?" She reached gently for him and found a large kitchen knife hidden in his robe. Without missing a beat she asked, "What are you doing with that?" She laughed benignly, as if she'd found a sponge or a bar of soap. "That doesn't belong there, silly. You know that. That's for cutting bread."

When she took the knife from him, he looked embarrassed and didn't resist. She put the knife away, ignoring the hammering in her chest.

"You must be hungry, dear. What are you in a mood for? Pancakes?" He stared at her blandly. "Should I make you some nice pancakes? Would you like that?"

He nodded mechanically. "Pancakes," he said, the knife totally forgotten.

Later, while Manley was watching television, Jean gathered up every knife, every sharp object—scissors, letter openers, knitting needles, and the like—and hid them in a chest in the basement. When she was done, she lowered herself heavily into a chair. Her hands were shaking violently, and her whole body trembled. The jumbled jabbering from the television provided a surreal background to the roiling emotions that raged through her.

Her imagination provided images of a knife sticking out of her back while Manley paced, oblivious. Had that been his purpose? To stab her? To seek revenge against the "boyfriend" he imagined she had? Was it for protection against an imagined enemy? Maybe he had thought to use it on himself. She didn't know.

She took a deep, shuddering breath. *Oh, God. Oh, God. Oh, God,* she prayed. The burden she had vowed to carry had grown far beyond what she had feared possible.

But how could she have envisioned that things would get this bad? She had known that Manley would become ill, that he would have problems, but she never anticipated that the daily struggle would be anything like this. She had no way of guessing that she would be caring for a toddler heading toward infancy. She never foresaw that she would be subsisting on so little sleep.

In all her life she had never heard of anyone going through this kind of experience. She knew there must be others like her who were struggling at this very moment with this terrible disease and who, like her, were losing touch with who they were.

After long minutes her heart had quieted, and she willed herself to stand. She would have to rush now. It was already 6:30, and she had to be at work at 8:00.

Steven had been going to classes only when he felt like it. He missed participating in sports, but he was comforted by remembering his outstanding athletic performances in happier days. Had things been different, he would have been thinking now about athletic scholarships and planning a try at professional baseball.

He wasn't bothered when boys and girls he knew were honored for academic achievement—he knew he was as smart or smarter than they were. As the school year drew to a close, old friends had been receiving acceptance letters from fancy colleges and universities, and he could easily have been one of them. As long as he knew it, what did he care if no one else did? He never doubted that he'd have his day, but his path was going to be different.

He found a job tending bar at a local place where Mike Fierro and he liked to hang out. Now his life had some structure. He had pocket money and an excuse to get away from home.

Home was where he was most helpless. He tried to assist his mother when that was possible, but his presence began to upset his father, as it had before his move to Maine. If Jean didn't ask him to stay home or do something special, he was gone until late into the night, then slept until noon.

Steven did his best to maintain a balance with his father. He had learned not to respond to Manley's irrational anger with more anger. If his mother seemed overwhelmed, Steven tried to distract Manley's attention. He tried to be sympathetic but firm and do what he imagined his father might have done if the situation were reversed. But Steven's patience was limited; he escaped when he could.

One thing he ran from was the sad, haunted look in his mother's eyes; another was the vacancy he saw in his father's face.

Jean realized that her son was suffering neglect, and she hated to have to decide between Manley and him, but she couldn't do it all. She barely knew Steven anymore. It hurt her to watch him growing hard and distant.

He seemed utterly indifferent to the fact that he would not graduate, and she could do nothing about it. She did not have the energy to impose her will on him. If she had the choice of getting tough with him or comforting him, she chose the gentler route, being honest about her feelings without alienating him. At least they could still laugh together, often about Manley's odd behavior. The laughter, more than anything, was a link between them.

Just before an appointment with Dr. Ellis, Jean received a shock when she stepped on a scale. In two weeks her weight had dropped fifteen pounds, leaving her a gaunt one hundred five. She had been eating plenty. Whenever she fed Manley, which was many times a day, she ate a little, too, so she expected to be heavier. Now, in Jay Ellis's office, an expression of consternation passed over the doctor's face when he looked at her. "Jean, what have you been doing to yourself? You look awful."

She blinked, stunned to silence by his bluntness.

"I'm not kidding," he said. "You look *old*."

Her lips quivered in anger. "What do you expect?" she snapped.

He went on talking, but she barely heard him through her haze of rage. She kept a tight rein on herself for the remainder of their meeting. As she drove home, however, she talked to herself, venting her fury. "How *dare* he! Who does he think he is?" Usually he was so positive, complimenting her about how well she was handling things. This time she felt insulted, and at that moment she hated him. "How could he be so *callous*?"

It took days for her to think rationally about Jay's concern. With Manley watching from the bathroom doorway, she studied herself in the mirror. Her face was haggard, her eyes sunken and dark. *He's right. I look awful. Like a zombie.* She bowed her head and closed her eyes. A small voice of self-preservation made itself known: *I have to take care of myself.*

The next morning she called up an exercise studio and inquired about classes. That evening she enlisted Laurie's help: Laurie would take Manley on Thursdays for a few hours after work so Jean could exercise.

Weeks later Jean saw Dr. Ellis again, and he commented that she looked better. She told him that she had been exercising and was trying to relax more.

"I couldn't stand you the last time we met," she told him. "You have no idea how furious I was."

"I think I have some idea."

"You had a purpose in saying those things to me, didn't you? Trying to get to me?"

"Yes," he admitted. "Frankly, I wasn't sure how you would react. You might have given up on yourself. It was a gamble, but someone had to shake you."

"Well, it worked." She smiled. "I suppose I should thank you."

He returned the smile in his thoughtful way. "I'm glad you could forgive me. I'd hate to lose you as a friend."

It was another day like hundreds before it. Manley had stormed out that summer morning, dressed in pajamas and slippers. She had run after him with his raincoat, which she finally convinced him to wear after a half an hour. For four hours they had walked through Clarksburg and North Adams. After their return to the house, he had eaten a big meal and settled down quietly with a word-puzzle book. He circled random groups of letters, and the page looked scribbled upon. Suddenly he exploded in a fit of temper.

Jean stood tensely in the kitchen, listening to her husband stomp around, then hit the bookshelves with his fists and yell unintelligibly. She had tried cajoling him and had offered him a sandwich and cookies, but he had thrown the food at her and continued his tirade. When she approached him, he swung at her. She tried to get out of his way, but he shoved her so hard she landed on the kitchen floor in a heap. Her husband's anger did not frighten her so long as he still seemed to know her. But increasingly now his eyes lacked any recognition, and that terrified her to the core.

A sound at the door behind her made her jump. Steven came in. He noted the fear and fatigue on her face. "What's going on?"

"He's on a rampage again."

Steven listened. Occasionally there was a crash as Manley struck out at some object or overturned a chair. Then there was a lull.

Manley unexpectedly came out of the den and toward the kitchen. The look in his eyes was murderous. Steven stepped in front of his mother.

"Hi, Dad!" he greeted in a friendly tone.

Manley said nothing. Then he whirled around and headed for the front door.

Steven followed. "Where you going, Dad? Want company?" He reached tentatively for his father's shoulder.

Manley whirled and struck his son's hand away forcefully. He was ready to attack. "No! No! No! Get!"

"Dad, what's the matter? I'm not trying to hurt you."

Manley turned and reached for the door, rattling it noisily, then finally got it open. He lurched outside.

"I'll go, Mom."

Jean collapsed into a chair at the kitchen table and lay her head on her arms. Jay Ellis had warned her that delusions and hallucinations were common among Alzheimer's victims. They tended to be suspicious and blamed the people close to them for whatever was going wrong. They might imagine someone was stealing money from them, hiding things from them, conspiring against them, even trying to hurt them. The paranoia, coupled with fragmented memory and waning comprehension, could concoct a totally distorted reality that seemed perfectly real. At times it was not unlike schizophrenia.

Jean had been gathering information on nursing homes and hospitals. She had even talked to people at the State Agency for Long-term Care in Springfield, Massachusetts, and they had scheduled Manley for an evaluation. She had been leaning toward nursing homes until she talked to Father Fay Sprague, who had highly recommended the Veterans Memorial Hospital in Northampton. The parish priest had been very impressed by the quality of individual care the staff provided for their patients.

Regardless of Dr. Ellis's warnings, she found it very difficult to face giving up her husband to the care of strangers. But now her back was to the wall.

Jean felt so threatened that she called Laurie from the kitchen phone after midnight. Only a few days had passed since Manley's last uncontrollable episode.

"I'm sorry to wake you," she said in tears. "I don't know what to do. I had to call someone for help."

"What's wrong, Mom? What happened?"

"Your father is just . . . well, more than I can handle. I hate to ask, but could Art come over and help me? Steven hasn't come home yet, and I don't feel safe."

Laurie said that Art would be right over.

Jean hung up the phone and tiptoed upstairs into Steven's room to get away from Manley's assaults. Then she listened for sounds of him. He was coming up the stairs after her.

Bravely she met him in the hallway. "Manley, dear, let me make you a snack. Come down to the kitchen. We can—"

Her words were cut off as Manley shoved her. She fell against the wall and lay there, whimpering and looking at her husband out of the corner of her eye. His face showed no recognition of her.

He advanced and stamped his foot. "Get!" he yelled. "Get!"

"Manley, please!"

He wavered.

She thought he would hit her, but he turned and paced. She cowered as he came at her again and swung his fist in her direction. The animallike sounds issuing from him were sheer, irrational rage. Then again he stalked away. This time he went into Steven's room.

Jean dashed for the stairs and flew down them before he came back. She ran into the master bedroom and locked the door behind her, panting with fear, then lay on the bed to wait.

Minutes later Art arrived, and Jean and he managed to give Manley a tranquilizer and get him into bed. After a while Manley had fallen asleep. Art slept on the couch, in case Jean needed him again.

The next day Jean called Dr. Everett about placing Manley at the Northampton Veterans Hospital.

"Take him down there, Jean, and let them evaluate Manley. I've found that's the best way. We'll avoid any complicated passing of records and red tape."

Jean discussed it with Laurie that night, and they decided to bring Manley to Northampton the following day. Manley's mood had improved somewhat, and Jean had increased his medication in the hope of keeping him quiet in the meantime.

Art got off work early and drove them all to the hospital. They announced themselves at the front desk and waited until Jean was ushered into the office of a social worker. Laurie and Art stayed with Manley in a waiting room full of vending machines and kept him occupied with snacks.

The social worker was a pleasant young man who listened intently to Jean's story. Then she introduced him to Laurie, Art, and Manley.

When Jean and the social worker were alone again, he gave his opinion that Manley should be admitted into the hospital; but the decision was not his. He arranged for the supervising doctor on duty to interview Manley.

The physician conferred briefly with the social worker, then spoke with Jean in her office. She had not heard of Alzheimer's disease but said she was familiar with the behavior of patients suffering from other forms of dementia.

The doctor thoroughly examined Manley with the help of two orderlies. Then she told Jean: "Your husband is qualified to be placed here, and I'll put him on our waiting list."

"I can't wait," Jean said desperately. "He's been violent."

"I'm afraid that's the best I can do for you, Mrs. Tyler."

"How long would I have to wait?"

"It could be as few as six months or as much as a year."

Jean caved in with a cry. "A year? I can't take it for another *day*. Don't you understand?"

"Of course I do. But dementia victims can be dealt with quite successfully, I assure you. And it's my experience that with proper medication and caution, your husband could be manageable for longer than you suppose."

Jean tried not to show her anger. Calmly she said, "Doctor, Manley is very strong and healthy. When he comes after me, I'm afraid for my life. He could kill me tonight."

"I feel for you, Mrs. Tyler. I advise you to stay out of his way and avoid doing things that provoke him."

Jean was speechless with frustration. *Do you think I'm a moron?* she wondered. In a shaky voice she pleaded, "The situation has gone beyond my avoiding him. He doesn't need to be provoked. His outbursts happen out of the blue most of the time. I've been caring for him for years. Maybe I've waited too long to seek help, but I wanted to give him as much time at home as possible." Tears were streaming from her eyes.

The doctor was silent, but her expression was set.

Jean got up. She would have liked to throttle this superior matron to let her know what it felt like. She started for the door.

The doctor followed her. "Avoid touching him so he won't be able to turn on you. Always have your back to a door so you can escape easily. When you need rest, lock yourself into your bedroom and sleep. That way, at least, you don't have to be worried about being assaulted while you're asleep. I'm sorry we can't do more for you, Mrs. Tyler, but you have to understand our position here."

Jean opened the door and slammed it shut behind her. *Stuff your position,* she thought. To Laurie and Art she said curtly, "They won't take him. Let's go."

Jean vented her feelings during the drive home, relating the doctor's ineffectual advice. "Can you believe it? Damn her!" Jean cursed hotly. "If I locked myself in the bedroom so I could get some sleep, Manley could wander unsupervised, doing whatever occurred to him! He could burn the house down, roam the countryside all night. Who knows what could happen? God, what a stupid woman!"

Jean was at a loss. Her foul mood had sent Manley into fretful ill-temper. He walked throughout the house impatiently. He peered distrustfully at Jean, Laurie, and Art as if trying to discern if they were friends or foes. He gnashed his teeth and made threatening growling sounds, with an occasional meaningless word of anguish. Jean was sure that only Art's presence prevented Manley from attacking her.

184

This has to be the worst point in my life, Jean thought.

Again with Art's help Jean gave Manley some tranquilizing medication.

Art tried to reassure his mother-in-law. "There's no way I'm going to leave you alone here tonight."

Laurie didn't stay long. She had to pick up Kate at an aunt's house. She kissed her mother and husband good-bye.

At about eight-thirty Jean and Art were able to get Manley to lie down and rest in the bedroom. They had some relief when he drifted off to sleep.

"We'd better rest while he's resting," Jean suggested. "I'm exhausted."

A little after midnight Manley began moving around. As she and Art tried to feed him in the kitchen, Jean sighed bitterly and said under her breath, "I can't stand it anymore. I really can't."

"I can't, either," Art responded, "and I've only been at it for a day or two. I can't imagine how you must feel."

Jean could not interest Manley in anything. She and Art kept an eye on him and tried to head off any problems.

Steven came home after 1:00 A.M. and helped them supervise his father.

At around 2:00 A.M. they persuaded Manley to lie down again. Before long they heard a rustling from the bedroom.

Jean held her head in her hands. "If you had a gun, I'd ask you to put me out of my misery," she said, an edge of hysteria to her tone.

Steven's voice tightened. "Mom, what are you talking about?"

"I mean it." But she looked at her son carefully. It was time for honesty. "I don't really want to commit suicide; I just don't know how much more I can take. I think I just want *out.*"

Manley, in his pajamas, opened the bedroom door. After seeing them in the den, he walked in the opposite direction.

"I thought the pills were supposed to make him sleepy," Art remarked.

"Sometimes they do," Jean replied. "But sometimes they don't. Don't ask me why."

Manley paced from the den to the living room and back again. They sat and listened.

"There's a lock on the bedroom door, right?" Art asked.

Jean looked at him as if he were crazy. "Yes."

"It locks from the inside?"

"Yes, why?"

"I'll turn it around."

"What?"

"I'll take out the doorknob and turn the lock around so you can lock it from the outside. Then maybe we can get some rest." He went to the basement for tools from Manley's workbench.

Art needed about twenty minutes to do the job. Meanwhile Jean fed Manley a sandwich, hopeful that the snack might make him drowsy. Then they put him to bed again and quietly locked him in.

Steven and Jean retired upstairs, and Art lay down on the couch in the den, close to the locked door of the master bedroom.

It took Art a long time to relax, but he did doze off. He awoke to a soft rattling of the door handle to the bedroom where Manley was. It was an eerie sound. The knob was being turned back and forth persistently but very calmly. The lack of urgency somehow made it creepier.

Art lay very still, listening, barely breathing. The sound went on for a long time but didn't become panicky or violent as he kept expecting it to. Finally it stopped.

Manley could easily break down the door if he wanted to, Art thought. *He could murder us all tonight.*

CHAPTER 21

Summer
1981

$\mathcal{L}$aurie called Jean's house at eight the next morning. Art told her that he and Jean had been up since six. No one had gotten much sleep, and Manley was once again wandering restlessly around the house. Steven, uncharacteristically, had gotten up early, too. Laurie said she would come over right away. It was obvious that something had changed, worsened.

She drove to Stonybrook Drive with Kate in the back seat. When she walked into the kitchen, her mother, husband, and brother were sitting at the table. Kate toddled to her father and then to her grandma, but neither could manage more than perfunctory enthusiasm for her.

Laurie could hear her father pacing and hitting the walls in the living room. She studied her mother with concern, and her heart ached. Jean looked as if she'd been crying all night. Her face revealed an inner collapse.

"Well, Mom, what do you think our plan of action should be today?"

"I don't know, I don't care, and frankly I don't give a good goddamn," she said in a lifeless monotone. "I have nothing left to give. I didn't know a person could be this tired and still be alive."

The words had a strong impact on Laurie; this was not her mother speaking. Steven was staring at Jean. Alarm had wiped the sleepiness from his face.

Laurie looked to her husband for some insight. Art gave her a grim look of someone who could not possibly describe the experience he and the others had lived through. Laurie felt as if the foundation of her world was collapsing, exposing the facts she worked so hard to conceal from herself. As her inner defenses toppled, she understood with painful clarity that her mother was on the brink of a breakdown. Her seemingly inexhaustible reserve of strength was used up. Something had to be done.

Laurie took a deep breath, stood, and walked carefully from the room, trying not to show the panic she felt.

She said hello to her father in the living room, but he looked right through her. She ran up the stairs to Steven's room and picked up the telephone, hating herself. How could she give up on her father? But she had to help her mother now, even if it was at her dad's expense. She dialed the number for Dr. Ellis's office, which she knew by heart. She told his secretary it was an emergency call about Jean Tyler, and he left a patient to take the call.

"Jay?" Laurie said when he picked up.

"Yes. What's wrong?"

"I've never seen my mother like this. I'm scared she's going to have a nervous breakdown. I don't think she can stand another day of this." She described what had happened at the veterans' hospital the day before and the evidently harrowing night Jean and Art had suffered.

"I was afraid it would come to this," Jay said. "It should never have gone on this long. Here's what you do. Get your father down to Berkshire Medical Center in Pittsfield. Can you be there by noon?"

"I think so."

"Good. I'll meet you in the main lobby. Bring pajamas, robe, and slippers—I'm going to get him admitted today."

"Thanks, Jay." She hung up and sat in silence on the edge of Steven's bed. *I'm sorry, Daddy,* she thought.

But now that she had taken action, her determination took over. She would not risk losing both parents. She picked up the phone again and dialed Father Fay Sprague. She told the priest what they were going through and the trouble they had had at the veterans' hospital. She was aware that he went there frequently and knew many of the doctors and administrators. She asked if he might be willing to intervene on the family's behalf and persuade the staff to accept her father.

Fay said he couldn't promise anything but would be glad to try. He also said he would try to talk to Congressman Silvio Conte.

Next Laurie got the number for Silvio Conte's regional office. The influential congressman was from North Adams and knew Manley and Father Fay and had long been a good friend to the DelNegro family.

She spoke to one of the congressman's aides and described

their dilemma. As Laurie detailed the situation, she felt herself growing stronger in her resolve. The aide told her that the congressman was in Washington, but he would try to get a call through to him. He would call her back in an hour.

Laurie was not finished. She got the number of the father of a friend who was active in the community and had connections to the American Legion and the Veterans of Foreign Wars. He was a kind and generous soul who cooked dinner for the homeless every Christmas at the American Legion Hall, and he and his wife donated their time at the Veterans Memorial Hospital. Laurie told him the entire story, emphasizing how desperate her mother's situation was. He promised to put a good word in for them with certain people he knew.

Laurie went downstairs. Her father was walking back and forth in the den. The threesome at the kitchen table had not moved.

After standing behind her mother, Laurie put a hand on Jean's shoulder and told her that Dr. Ellis had instructed them to meet him at Berkshire Medical Center in Pittsfield.

Jean tilted her head back wearily and looked for a long moment into her daughter's eyes.

"Okay." She took Laurie's hand in her own and squeezed it, closing her eyes and inhaling deeply.

"It's going to be okay, Mom," Laurie said.

As they made preparations, the phone rang. It was the congressman's aide. He said that Silvio Conte remembered Manley and would be happy to contact the hospital on the family's behalf. Laurie thanked him warmly.

She and her mother drove Manley to Pittsfield where Dr. Ellis met them. He had already made preliminary arrangements for Manley's admittance. He complied without a struggle as they settled him into his room.

Jay spoke briefly to Jean and Laurie before they left the hospital. "As far as I'm concerned, Manley is not going home anymore. I can't tell you what to do, but I believe that you've done far, far more than could be expected for his comfort and peace of mind. It's time for him to be cared for by trained professionals."

In a monotone Jean surrendered. "I guess you're right, Jay. I'm at my wit's end."

"That's this year's understatement. You need a rest."

In the car on the way home she reflected on what Jay had said. *At least he didn't say: "I told you so,"* she realized. *He very easily could have.*

Dr. Ellis enlisted a psychiatrist to evaluate Manley's mental status. Manley was more likely to be admitted to the veterans' hospital if his behavior was determined to be violent, and he made things easy because on his first day at Berkshire Medical Center he bit a nurse who was trying to undress him.

In her calls to the veterans' hospital, Jean was advised that Manley's best chance to be admitted immediately would be on a so-called ten-day paper, or a temporary stay of ten days. Once he was there, she was told, he would be evaluated by staff. If he was already under their care, it might be easier to keep him there permanently.

As a result Jean asked that he be admitted under a ten-day paper.

By Manley's third day at BMC, Jean was notified that he would be accepted in Northampton for the ten-day stay. She had no way of knowing which of the several people Laurie contacted had made the difference in getting him admitted.

Manley was taken by ambulance to Northampton and placed in the psychiatric ward at Veterans Memorial Hospital. Jean was advised not to visit him for a few days; it was standard operating procedure, allowing the hospital staff to evaluate a patient on their own.

Manley had been admitted to BMC on 1 July. With the Fourth of July coming up, Laurie and Art tried to talk Jean into vacationing with them in northern Vermont. She declined that and other invitations to cookouts and parties. She felt terrible; she was far from ready to socialize.

Being in an empty house without the constant pressure of caring for Manley came as a shock to her system. As the tension eased, physical pain set in. She had been living in a state of unrelenting exhaustion, with her body unable to relax, for so long, that when the pressure subsided, she ached everywhere. The pain lasted for days as the strains that had kept her in knots slowly eased.

For a change she could sleep, but it was fitful and fretful. Sleeping undisturbed and deeply was something else she had to relearn. While friends and family celebrated the Fourth of July, she stayed home alone, still enveloped by exhaustion, tension, and fear.

Her emotions fluctuated wildly as she alternately felt relieved that Manley was in a good place and guilty that she had not been able to hang on longer. She also feared what would happen if she was forced to bring her husband home after the ten days expired. She cried a lot.

She called the hospital every day to ask about Manley and to check if the staff understood his problems. She wondered if they would experience the same difficulties that the nurses at North Adams Regional Hospital had had. But she was assured that everything was under control.

After Manley's fifth day at the facility, Jean was permitted to visit him. His face lit up when he saw her. She hugged him hard and shed a few tears. He seemed composed and calm, a great improvement over the craziness of his last weeks at home. Perhaps, she thought, these people *did* know what they were doing, and perhaps it *was* better for him to be there now. She was very impressed with the pleasant staff and their sensitivity toward her. The hospital ran very efficiently and was not nearly as depressing as she had expected.

When it was time for her to leave, Manley became upset. A nurse asked Jean to come back into the room and sit with Manley for a while longer, so she could try something that usually worked in such instances.

Once Manley became calm again, the nurse distracted him, saying, "Come, Manley, let's walk down to the end of the ward."

This was obviously a routine he had become used to, and he got up and allowed himself to be led toward the door. When his back turned, the nurse motioned for Jean to leave. She went the opposite direction but stayed to watch from a hidden vantage point to see if he would get upset again. She could see, however, that he had completely forgotten about her. With a sigh she left.

When the ten days of Manley's temporary stay had passed, Jean met with the no-nonsense social worker in charge of his ward.

"Your husband's ten-day term is up, and you will have to take him home again," the woman said. "If you would be so good as to sign these release papers? . . ."

Jean had been coached for this crucial meeting by someone familiar with the institution's procedures. She said firmly, "I can't handle him."

"I'm afraid you'll have to. I'm sure the supervising physician informed you that there is a waiting list for permanent places here. You husband's turn may not come up for some time."

It was the hardest thing she had ever done, but Jean repeated what she had to say. "No. I can't take him. He's in your hands."

"Are you saying, Mrs. Tyler, that we should just let him loose on the street? That you wash your hands of him?" She looked outraged.

"That's what I'm saying," Jean confirmed. "You've got him. He's your responsibility now. I can't deal with him anymore." She waited and clamped her jaw shut so she wouldn't say: *He's my husband, the only man I've ever loved. Of course I can take care of him.* For a long moment silence prevailed. The tension was palpable in this contest of wills.

Then the social worker said, "Well, if that's the way you feel, I guess we have no choice in the matter." Then she allowed herself a small smile.

Jean returned it knowingly. "Thank you," she said, meaning it from the bottom of her heart.

Manley had a new home.

Part
III

CHAPTER 22

Fall
1981

*S*teven Tyler had not graduated with his class in the spring of 1981, but once he was free of the tethers of his high school, he began to wonder about his future. He did not worry the way his mother did. She had tearfully pleaded with him to salvage his life before it was too late. She was in constant fear that he'd get seriously hurt or in trouble with the law, since she had inklings of the wild life he'd been leading.

In June, just a week before his father was placed in the veterans' hospital, Steven had made an appointment with the dean of admissions at North Adams State College. During the interview, Steven boldly explained what had happened to his family and him. He described how he had been a straight-A student until the onset of his father's illness, but he was confident that he could perform college work. He asked to be admitted to the college despite his poor record.

The dean was impressed with Steven's forthrightness and intelligence. He had also heard of Manley Tyler, a well-known alumnus of North Adams State College. After the dean studied Steven's record, he decided to approve his acceptance, provided the young man earned a high-school equivalency diploma.

Steven had attended a class at Berkshire Community College in Pittsfield to earn his diploma over the summer. He easily passed the requirements.

Now, with school about to begin, Jean talked to him about his plans. Since she could hardly afford tuition, she suggested that he apply to Berkshire Community College, which was less expensive than North Adams State. Steven did so and was accepted into a liberal-arts program.

To help ease the financial burden, Steven worked as an aide at a local nursing home.

Steven wanted to do the right things for his mother's sake, but he didn't know what he wanted. His only enjoyment was hanging out with his drinking buddies; alcohol made him feel human. He didn't live his life so much as he allowed it to carry him along. He wandered through the forested mountains around Clarksburg. The woods were the one place he felt he belonged. He had a few favorite spots where he would build a small fire if it was cold. He spent hours staring into the flames, thinking about his future.

His mother was immersed in an ongoing frenzy of ceaseless activity, and Steven was proud of her astonishing drive. But for himself there seemed to be no clear-cut path. His father's illness had been suffocating him for as long as he could remember. Steven's very identity was caught up in wrestling with understanding Manley's misfortune.

Life was better now that his father was out of the house. Manley seemed calmer, and his disapproval of Steven was gone for the most part. The young man was glad for that.

As Jean's tensions subsided, the pain that had raged like a cleansing fire in her body gradually faded. At last she was able to rest, but she endured other tortures. Guilt and doubt continued to assail her. She was plagued by the feeling that she should have sought temporary hospitalization for Manley, rather than a permanent accommodation.

Manley didn't seem nearly so threatening since he'd been institutionalized. Perhaps his violence had been a passing thing? . . . Might it have been triggered by something she did or did not do? If so, then she had not done a very good job of caring for him.

She punished herself with the recurring thought that *she* was responsible for the well-being of her husband. But she had given up and passed his care to someone else. It didn't matter if she'd had no choice. Self-loathing ate at her like acid.

She visited Manley four or five days a week and got to know the scenery on the fifty-mile ride between North Adams and Northampton by heart. Dr. Ellis advised her to go less often and reduce her strain, but she ignored him because Manley was always happy to see her.

He had been moved from the psychiatric ward to D Annex, which was a closed, uncrowded, well-supervised area for long-term patients, some of whom exhibited dementing illness. His bed was one of four in a large, open room. As Jean became acquainted with the staff, she was highly impressed by their personal commitment, training, and experience. The professionals had high standards, yet there was an air of spirited and friendly cooperation. Manley was well-groomed at all times and was given considerable attention by orderlies, nurses, and doctors every day. They got to know him quickly, and Jean was kept apprised of his behavior.

She could not imagine better care; the staff genuinely liked Manley, and to Jean's relief, he seemed to like them. It surprised her that he responded so positively.

Though she felt good about the quality of care Manley was receiving, the hollowness inside her persisted. Often during the hour-long ride to Northampton she broke down and cried, wallowing helplessly in haunting memories and self-accusation.

She had gone back to working full-time at Lamb Printing, but financial pressures were unrelenting. The car needed repairs every month, and gasoline became a big expense.

It had been ten years since Manley's last days as an educator—a decade that felt like a lifetime. The world had gradually turned joyless, barely worth living in. But she persevered with steely stoicism. She wondered often about other families who were going through comparable experiences. It occurred to Jean that such caregivers could benefit from the help of someone who had already lived through the horror.

Though she'd been very fortunate to have Dr. Ellis's support, even his expertise had not adequately prepared her for dealing with Manley. She had learned it all the hard way, through trial and error. *How many are living through that hell this very moment,* she wondered, *totally alone in their hardship, completely misunderstood by friends and community, with their lives coming undone?*

She had found out that no awareness of such suffering existed in the community. Because of public and professional ignorance, the plight of Alzheimer patients' households remained a secret. Because of what had happened to her family in past years, she had lost her naive trust in life and society. She was not the person she used to be.

Jean wanted to express her gratitude to the many people who had helped her in getting Manley situated and who had lent a hand or sympathetic ear during the years of her ordeal.

She knew no words could ever convey the depth of her feelings to Manley's aunt Charlotte, without whose daily uncomplaining sacrifice Jean could not have functioned at all. Charlotte Exford had given her time and energy day after day without thought for repayment.

Jean knew she'd have to thank Jay Ellis in person. When Manley had been at Northampton for a month, Jean paid the neurologist a visit.

"I couldn't have made it without you," she told him.

"Are you kidding? I did nothing," he responded. "You did it all."

"Maybe you don't realize it, Jay, but just having someone who understood what I was talking about helped to get me through. People just can't comprehend the problems unless they've experienced them personally."

"But I just know about Alzheimer's from a neurological standpoint."

"You cared, and that meant more than you know. There's got to be something I can do for other people living through it now. You come into contact with Alzheimer's cases. When you hear of other victims, I'd appreciate your giving me the names of the caregivers. Maybe I can help them."

Jay was taken aback. "That is *not* a good idea," he said firmly. "You barely survived your own experience. You're lucky you didn't have a physical or emotional breakdown."

"But that's what I mean," she replied earnestly. "I could warn families about what is going to happen and help them avoid what it did to me." She stared past him, lost in thought for a moment, recalling the nightmarish blur of the past decade. "I made a lot of mistakes and kidded myself, didn't I? I didn't want to see the truth, hoping that by not acknowledging it, it would go away. My blindness may have made things worse for Steven and Laurie."

"I can't believe you want to do this." Jay studied her from across his desk.

A troubled look flitted across Jean's features. "It bothers me to know that someone out there is going through the same hell right now. A few words of encouragement or advice could make such a difference."

"That's true." The young doctor, resigned to her decision, leaned back in his chair. "But I urge you to give it a lot of thought before you take on any additional burdens."

"I will. But I have too much time to think now. I want to do something positive about this lousy disease."

That week Jean read an article in the *Berkshire Eagle* about a workshop concerned with the problems of the elderly. The article mentioned Elizabeth Powers, who described her mother's aberrant behavior. The sixty-eight-year-old woman had been confused at Elizabeth's wedding reception, thinking that she was at her own high-school reunion decades before. The distraught young bride said her mother had Alzheimer's disease, of which no one had heard. She and her father didn't know what they were going to do or where to turn for help.

The next day Jean called Elder Services of Berkshire County, which had sponsored the workshop, and requested and received Elizabeth Powers's work number. Jean introduced herself over the phone and described a few of her own experiences with Manley. Then she asked if she could be of any help, perhaps just to listen. Liz began to cry, profoundly moved that someone had sought her out. Jean invited Liz to her house, and the woman accepted and asked if she might bring her father.

That week Liz and her father, Tom Powers, came to Clarksburg and confided what they had been going through. It sounded all too familiar to Jean. Once father and daughter started talking about their plight, floodgates of emotion opened.

Tom lived with his wife, Elaine, and was assuming the responsibility for her care; Liz, who lived fifteen miles away, helped out four or five days a week.

Liz described her mother's wandering, which usually followed a period of anger. "She'll become angry over nothing—a water spot on a glass, for instance. Then she'll say that she is leaving and will pack her bags. She doesn't know where she is going, but she'll pack everything she'd need for a trip. She'll sneak out when I'm in another part of the house. Sometimes she says that she wants to go home, not realizing that she already is at home."

Jean listened quietly about Elaine's frequent periods of melancholy and failed memory.

"Much of the time," Liz said sadly, "she doesn't know that I'm her daughter."

They talked for hours. Jean heard them out, then described her own feelings. She could see that it was good for Tom and Liz to talk; despair held a little less sting when shared. The three even laughed together.

Jean discussed her intention of organizing informal gatherings for Alzheimer's caregivers. Liz was interested in helping.

When they said good-bye, Jean was certain that their talk had been helpful. Now, at least, Tom and Liz knew someone to call if they wanted to talk or ask advice.

In the next week Jay Ellis gave Jean the phone number of a caregiver. Jean, Liz, Tom, and the new woman met at the Elder Services headquarters with a representative of that organization and discussed how to proceed with forming a support group. The Elder Services representative was very encouraging but suggested that the Alzheimer's group should function separately from Elder Services to avoid legal complications.

Jean and Liz placed advertisements in the North Adams *Transcript* as well as the Pittsfield *Berkshire Eagle,* announcing the formation of their support group.

Most responses came from the Pittsfield area, so Jean traveled the twenty miles to visit the callers' homes. Sometimes a few people gathered at Liz's house.

By September, with the help of Elder Services of Berkshire County, Jean obtained permission from First Agricultural Bank in Pittsfield to use a conference room for the first meeting of the support group. More than a dozen people attended.

Jean felt self-conscious speaking to the group and thought how ironic it was that Manley had been a natural leader. But she plodded ahead. Once she began telling about what she had gone through, others began to do the same, talking openly and with growing trust.

For many members this was the first time they could describe what they were going through to someone who really understood. With great intensity they vented anger and frustration and confusion. Shame was prevalent because of archaic attitudes toward anything that sounded like a mental disorder. People connected deeply with each other and often shed tears that had been stanched for too long or vented anger long denied. Of greatest value was the members' understanding that they weren't alone.

Jean stressed the importance of laughing and fondly recalled her leaning on the indomitable Angie Potter. In a small way the self-help group fought the impact of hopelessness, which eroded the strength and morale of Alzheimer's caregivers.

Between monthly meetings Jean privately contacted each member by phone or at their home, listening to their personal struggles and making suggestions. She encouraged them to call her at home in the evenings if they wished to.

Each family, she learned, had its own unique problems. Caregiving was physically strenuous, and some caregivers were so elderly that commonplace problems became difficult. Caregivers might have their own serious ailments. But the worst problem had to do with emotions, loneliness being the worst. Jean knew how she herself would have welcomed the existence of such a group a few years before.

Jean reflected about what she was doing. She had been right to follow this path. Each time she acted as group leader, the role felt more comfortable. Commiserating smiles and renewed strength in her new acquaintances made Jean feel that she had finally struck a blow against the disease that had plunged her life into chaos.

Laurie went with Jean to a few meetings. She was filled with admiration and amazement at what her mother was doing. *How could she do this after what she's been through? She has such strength!*

Laurie was shocked by how angry she felt at the meetings. The caregivers and the Alzheimer's victims were a generation older than her parents. *Why did Dad have to get it when he was so young?* she wondered. It wasn't fair!

At the end of one meeting a woman came up to Jean. "I can't tell you how grateful I am that you're doing this," Laurie heard her say. The woman's sad eyes were eloquent with feeling. "I've lost touch with all my friends and family. No one understands. I've been so alone." She managed a small, brave smile. "Now I feel part of the human race again."

Nineteen eighty-one had been a whirlwind for Jean. After Manley was hospitalized, the support group engaged all her spare time and energy. The endeavor, which Jean had thought would be an occasional thing, turned into a full-time activity. Her phone never stopped ringing.

Steven bought his mother an answering machine so she wouldn't miss any calls.

Jean was astounded by how many people were afflicted by Alzheimer's disease in her local area, which was not densely populated. She had never imagined that so many were suffering what she had suffered. Alzheimer's was just beginning to enter the consciousness of society. The medical community as well as the general public were slowly becoming acquainted with it, chiefly through a few cases that made headlines in the national media: Norman Rockwell, the famous Massachusetts illustrator, had died of it in 1978. Rita Hayworth was diagnosed in 1979. Reports of the movie star's strange behavior shocked the public. How sad that the beautiful actress, a darling of the forties, had come to such an ignominious end.

The Alzheimer's support group continued to draw more people through ads and word-of-mouth communication. Dr. Ellis sent more people to Jean, also. She continued to visit many members in their homes because monthly meetings were not always adequate to address the morass of problems to be faced in some families.

She never begrudged anyone her time; helping others made her feel good about herself, and it kept her busy—she didn't want time to think. She could subjugate her own problems in the more urgent dilemmas of the group members.

Jean was surprised to find that the group members didn't want her to show weakness. If she tried to vent her frustrations or negative emotions, they wouldn't accept it. For some reason they had decided that she, as leader, belonged in a separate category. As she had done for so long, she had to continue to be strong for others.

She still met regularly with Jay Ellis for her own "therapy." He asked if young interns might sit in, and Jean assented. The new doctors listened and learned from her growing wealth of knowledge about the stresses and complexities of caregiving.

She and other members decided to invite professionals to speak to the group on specific areas of expertise: legal and medical matters, obtaining government assistance, the advantages of nursing homes and hospitals, and so on.

Dr. Ellis was their first speaker. Over forty people were in attendance. He gave a thorough discourse on Alzheimer's disease from a neurologist's perspective, plus his own growing insights on the difficult task of caregiving. He was especially interested in dispelling popular misconceptions about the dementing illness.

"One thing I can't emphasize enough," he said, "is that Alzheimer's is not caused by hardening of the arteries in the brain. Contrary to what was once believed, arteriosclerosis has nothing to do with it. Alzheimer's may be caused by hereditary factors, an obscure virus, some exotic poison, a combination of things, or none of the above. The truth is we have no idea what causes it—not a clue . . . not yet."

Afterward Jay answered many questions. When the meeting broke up that night, Jean thanked him for his participation.

"I didn't expect such a crowd," he responded. "You've really jumped into this with both feet." He chuckled quietly. "Jean, I was wrong about this undertaking: You look more alive than I've seen you looking in a long time.''

Driving home that night was a passage in deafening silence, but conversations from the past few days replayed in Jean's mind.

Life continues to barrel along, she thought, *and the unthinkable has happened. I can speak to you, Manley, but I must answer for you, too. How long ago it seems that I was your supportive wife, your closest friend. We had such good times, such fun. Rides through the countryside were celebrations then.*

She steered her car through the night. Dead, dry leaves tumbled across her path, blown by gusts that buffeted her car. It was a small leap to imagine herself as the only person in the world who was out tonight. When she arrived home, the turn of her key in her front door lock had an empty sound of finality. The bustle and chatter of better days had gone forever.

She stepped into her dark house, and the silence took hold. It was after eleven. Something about the quiet made her hurry as she got ready for bed.

She turned out the light on the nightstand, sighed, and gave herself up to exhaustion. Sleep eluded her, however. She was numbed by crushing loneliness. The success of this night's meeting accentuated Manley's absence.

Lying alone in the dark, she began to face the true enormity of losing him. Never would she again share with him. She faced the rest of her days as a solitary woman. A wave of emotion caught her. For the first time in weeks she gave in to choking sobs.

A memory found its way, unbidden, to her consciousness: It was a wonderful day in 1970. She and Manley and another couple had gone to Saratoga, New York, during the late-summer horse-racing season. Manley had left Jean and the others to buy some sandwiches. When he returned, carrying the tray of food, Jean watched him come up the crowded steps, dodging people surging around him. As he approached he smiled dazzlingly, sending a familiar thrill through her. *We've been married eighteen years,* she had thought, *yet he's as handsome as the first day I saw him. His physical beauty matches the beauty of his inner spirit. What a lucky woman I am to be married to such a jewel of a man! If I had my choice of every man in the world, I would still pick Manley.*

Now she thought: *You are dying by degrees, darling, but I'll never ever forget what we were together. Nothing can ever kill that.*

203

Spring – Summer 1982

*J*ean was surprised to hear from Brent Filson, a journalist who
asked to interview her for a two-part article on Alzheimer's disease. It would appear in the "Berkshire Sampler," the weekend
magazine of the *Berkshire Eagle*. The idea of her very personal
story being published in a newspaper repelled Jean. Brent asked her
to think about it; he would wait to hear from her.

She agonized over her decision for a week and asked Laurie
and Angie for their opinions. Laurie had no objections and said that
it would have been the kind of thing her father would do.

Angie also was positive about it. "Will it bother you to have
people reading about you?" she asked.

"I never counted on making Manley's personal ordeal so public."

"What do you think Manley would want you to do?"

"Laurie thinks he would want me to do it. It was his way to
shed light on the truth whenever he could."

"It would help bring more people forward, wouldn't it?"

Jean had to agree. She decided to sacrifice her privacy. Brent
interviewed Jean, Liz Powers, and Dr. Ellis. The young writer even
visited Manley in Northampton and met with Laurie and Steven.

The articles proved thorough and informative. Jean's phone
number was included for people who wished to contact her about
the support group.

In the weeks after the articles were published, Jean's phone
rang off the hook. She was taken aback by the extent of the
response, never having dreamed that so many people had been
touched by Alzheimer's disease. While she had been caring for

Manley at home, she felt as if she was the only caregiver in the county.

One of the elderly members of Jean's support group had attended a forum on human services in Springfield, Massachusetts, and met Dr. Joan Hyde, executive director of the eastern Massachusetts chapter of Alzheimer's Disease and Related Disorders Association. The ADRDA was a growing national organization assisting caregivers of people with Alzheimer's and other dementing illnesses. Through Jean's elderly acquaintance, Joan Hyde found out about the Berkshire County self-help group. Dr. Hyde gave her number to the elderly man with instructions that Jean Tyler should call her in Boston.

Jean and Dr. Hyde had a long talk. Jean had never heard of ADRDA and was pleased to learn of its existence. Joan Hyde, in turn, was surprised and pleased to learn about Jean's activities in the often-overlooked far-western part of the state. She gave Jean her home phone number and urged her to call for information or advice.

Thus Jean became aware that a growing network of support activity was crisscrossing the nation. She also learned that what she had been doing during support meetings was called *facilitating*.

In the weeks that followed, Joan sent Jean booklets and brochures from ADRDA and other sources on specific aspects of the dilemma of caring for an Alzheimer's victim. The doctor also recommended knowledgeable people in that part of the state who might speak to the Alzheimer's group in Pittsfield.

Much to Jean's chagrin, Steven dropped out of college after one semester and put more time into his late-night drinking. It was a daily battle to get him out of bed in the morning.

Jean sought help from every quarter. Dr. Bill Everett suggested counseling, and to please his mother, Steven went to see a psychologist. He spent a long hour answering questions and trying to describe his thoughts. At the session's end the therapist told Steven that he thought the young man was as emotionally healthy as could be expected under the circumstances.

Early in 1982 Steven found a full-time job as an installer for a national company that offered cable television in North Adams and Williamstown. He earned money and partied and did not shrink from fistfights. His mother worried that she'd get a call from the police saying that he was in jail, but Steven was adamant about being allowed to live his own life.

Meanwhile, Art and Laurie and six other small business owners created an indoor shopping mall in North Adams. Art and Laurie operated a sporting-goods store, and they worked there in shifts.

Laurie, pregnant again, had her hands full working at the fledgling shop, taking care of two-year-old Kate, and maintaining their home. Art's time was divided between the mini-mall and his mother's ski-specialty shop. He also coached football, officiated at softball games, and tended bar two nights a week.

Laurie and Art frequently visited Manley with Jean. Katie usually went, too. The little girl and Manley got along famously, and such visits had a party atmosphere. They would all walk with Manley to the lounge, which had a piano and television. They bought cookies or other snacks and fed him his beloved junk food.

His speech had noticeably worsened. He would trip over a word and repeat it in a kind of mental stutter. He was usually equable, but sometimes his eyes clouded with the sad awareness that he was ill, and he would be unhappy. When it was time for the family to go home, Manley would watch the departure as if he was losing that which was most precious to him but could do nothing about it.

Laurie continued to resist accepting the inevitable. She remained optimistic that her father might still recover. When she was at his side, she maintained a steady monologue for his benefit, hopeful that her words would have a healing effect.

Persistent guilt ate at her that she had not done as much as her mother and brother to help her father. Jean tried to allay these feelings, saying that Laurie had more than enough to deal with at home. But the young woman had high expectations for herself and couldn't help but feel that she should have done more.

"What more could you have done, Laur?" Jean would ask.

"I don't know, Mom. Something."

"You did plenty. You were out of the house, married, then you had Kate. A person can only do so much. I see similar guilt and self-doubt in the support-group people. Good people never feel as if they've done enough. They're always criticizing themselves. Don't do it to yourself, Laurie."

Although Jean was working full-time, her debts totaled over four thousand dollars. The savings that Manley and she had set aside before his resignation as principal had been eaten up years before, during the six-month wait for his disability payments from Social Security. The social-security disability and Jean's wages combined were not enough to keep up with her living expenses, let alone to clear her of debt. The mortgage had to be paid, of course, as well as food bills, clothing, utilities, and a dozen other odds and ends, not least of which was an old and failing car. She felt she was always on a tightrope, paying a little here and there so her creditors wouldn't initiate legal action. It was humiliating for her.

In the spring of 1982 she was informed by her mechanic that her Ford Fairmont station wagon needed a new engine. Fortunately, a friend of the family found an engine in a junkyard and installed it for a very modest three hundred dollars. But the car was still unreliable, and she needed it to travel to Northampton several times a week as well as to her support-group meetings and on visits to members' homes. She needed a new car.

She had been thinking about selling the house. Since Manley no longer lived there, she was not attached to it anymore, and she certainly didn't need the space—Steven would not be living with her much longer. After serious consideration, she came to a decision. She contacted a real-estate broker and had her house put on the market.

By June of 1982 it was sold. Finally she could pay off all her debts. She also contributed generously to Alzheimer's disease research. She did not have so much money from the sale of the house to warrant it under normal circumstances, but she felt that part of the money was Manley's, and what better place to donate than to fight the disease that was killing him?

She traded in the station wagon and purchased a new Subaru. She had come to suspect that Steven was rough on cars, so she bought him a used Toyota Corona to keep him away from her own car.

While looking for a place to live, Jean stayed with Laurie and Art, then moved into a very comfortable apartment in an old house in the center of North Adams. Freedom from money worries gave her the flexibility to make long-distance calls to the Massachusetts chapter of ADRDA in Boston and toll calls to members of the Alzheimer's self-help group.

Because the network had swelled to over sixty participants and was at the point of being unmanageable, Jean started another group in Williamstown with the help of Mary Coury, an energetic member of the Pittsfield organization. Mary made calls, mailed literature, and helped in fund-raising activities. Jean facilitated those support-group meetings as well, but eventually another active member, Esther Tauber, offered to take over.

207

Fund-raising became an all-important activity. Although Jean knew that the meetings were the backbone of support, members still had to return home to face the same situation. A need existed for more than mere talk; she wanted to accomplish tangible things—to help the most financially needy and obtain professional help in various areas. She and other volunteers would leave cards telling of their meetings in doctor's offices, hospitals, and funeral homes. Printing cards and literature for distribution cost money.

They tried a variety of activities to raise money: They held tag sales and bake sales; they persuaded a local food chain to contribute funds. If a shopper obtained a certain card, the food store would donate a percentage of its receipts to the Alzheimer's support group. Family members and friends at memorial services of deceased Alzheimer's victims also contributed generously.

The constant activity between her job and the support work kept despair at bay; the only time she couldn't avoid it was when she was with Manley.

CHAPTER 24

Early 1983

After Christmas the company for which Steven worked offered him a position in San Francisco. In January of 1983, he drove cross-country in one of four company vans. Distancing himself from home allowed Steven some clarity about who he was, and life held surprises for him.

At work Steven met a fellow who played semiprofessional baseball for a double-A team. Steven questioned him about his team, Las Aguilas, which meant the Eagles. The fellow mentioned that they needed pitchers.

The following week Steven went to the ballpark after work and was introduced to the team manager. Even though Steven still had on his work boots, the manager sent him to the mound. He pitched to a player taking batting practice. Steven had control and confidence. The manager asked him to return the next day for a real tryout.

Steven made the team. It was thrilling to be on a baseball diamond again. He worked into it gradually, happy that he hadn't lost his touch. He had not forgotten the fastball, the slow curve, or the knuckleball that his father had taught him so many years before. In a couple of weeks his fastball was clocked at eighty-five miles an hour. He was soon made a starter. He practiced after work and earned fifty dollars for every day that he showed up at the ballpark.

His teammates were all Mexican-Americans. They kidded him about being the "token white guy." It didn't bother Steven; he clowned with them, and his good humor won them over. They accepted him easily, and he was genuinely happy with the team.

Steven finished the remainder of the season, winning eight games with no losses. His team took second place in the standings. He felt as if a missing part of himself had been restored.

The Alzheimer's support group in Pittsfield grew until the bank's conference room could not accommodate the gathering. The meetings moved to the larger Berkshire Rehabilitation Center down the street.

Besides facilitating the support groups and filling the myriad needs that went along with it, Jean initiated a host of other new activities connected with Alzheimer's disease. With the help of a local service organization, the support group conducted a day-long conference on Alzheimer's disease at Berkshire Community College. Another project was to write a proposal for starting an exclusively Alzheimer's wing at a local nursing home, whose owner was willing.

When she had a moment to view herself objectively, Jean was surprised by her abilities. She learned as she went. She had never had any organizational or managerial experience—she'd been a wife and mother most of her life. Her jobs had not prepared her adequately. But she saw what had to be done, and she bulled ahead, enlisting any possible cooperation and assistance along the way.

Jean and other members tried every available method of disseminating their information to the community. In her opinion, educating the public was an extremely important part of battling the disease. The more people who knew the truth about Alzheimer's, the easier it would become for caregivers to find help in the community. Teachers, social workers, police, and local government operatives at every level needed to understand the nature of the illness and the unique stresses it created within families.

Jean remained in touch with the eastern Massachusetts chapter of ADRDA. Dr. Joan Hyde sent her the latest literature and news about research. She also continued to recommend a number of experts who came to speak to the Pittsfield and Williamstown support groups. One such speaker was Joan's superior, Dr. F. Marott Sinex, president of the eastern Massachusetts chapter of the ADRDA and head of the biochemistry department of Boston University Medical School. Jean arranged for Dr. Sinex to speak at Berkshire Medical Center instead of at their usual meeting place.

Two hours before he was scheduled to speak, Jean and Dr. Sinex had dinner in a restaurant. He wanted to know about her and how she was doing as leader of the fledgling support group. From him she learned more about ADRDA and the Boston chapter. They enthusiastically discussed their aims and strategies for surmounting obstacles and became so involved with their conversation that they were late getting to BMC for his talk.

A sizable audience had gathered. The doctor discussed the disease, the challenges of reaching people who needed help, and his experience with caregivers' problems and strategies.

After the meeting, Dr. Sinex told Jean that he was pleasantly surprised at the turnout; he had not expected such a strong organization in a rural area.

The following week Joan Hyde called and said, "Marott was really impressed with you, Jean. He couldn't praise you enough. He told me: 'Not only can Jean Tyler handle western Massachusetts, she could handle the whole East Coast if we let her.'"

"Who, me?" Jean asked, flabbergasted.

"Yes, you," Joan said, laughing.

A month later Jean learned that she had been appointed to sit on the board of directors of the ADRDA chapter in Boston. They wanted her involved more directly with ADRDA if she was willing. Again, she had to ask herself: *Who me?*

But she certainly was willing. She made regular trips to Boston for the quarterly meetings and became acquainted with the procedures of ADRDA. She was introduced to many people from eastern Massachusetts.

Jean's activities filled her time. When she stopped to think about it, she was amazed at how busy she was. It was just as well, because her visits to Northampton to see Manley grew more painful as time passed.

The effect of his brain deterioration had confined him to bed much of the time. He looked more and more aged. Still, he never failed to respond to her. He didn't exhibit the total lack of recognition she had feared might occur. His eyes always lit up when she came into his room.

To see him slowly but surely dying was almost more than she could bear. It was the cruelest torture she could imagine. Manley was condemned to live like this, dying by degrees, and she was sentenced to watch.

Jean's heart felt like a heavy brick in her chest. She never showed her anguish when she was with Manley. She wanted him to perceive only the warmth and normalcy he had always known with her, no matter what. But more than once she left him and went into the woman's room, put a towel into her mouth, and screamed into it.

She preferred the exhausting labor of her activities with Alzheimer's to a visit with her husband; that fact intensified the guilt she hadn't shaken since having placed him in the hospital. There were times when she set out for Northampton, dreading it more and more as she drove nearer, until she could barely continue.

On one such day she had driven more than halfway to the hospital when she suddenly had to stop the car at the side of the road. She turned off the ignition and closed her eyes. *It's something I have to do. But I don't want to go. I just don't want to go. I'm sorry, Manley. I just can't face it today. Please forgive me.* She started the car and turned it around. Her feeling of relief as she drove home was marred, of course, by powerful guilt.

CHAPTER 25

Late 1983 –
Early 1984

*I*n the fall Steven missed his mother, sister, and the New England change of seasons. He couldn't imagine spending Christmas on the West Coast. He knew he had to go home; he had to be part of the family again.

In December, halfway through his second baseball season, he returned to North Adams just in time for Christmas.

Jean noticed a promising change in Steven. He was more willing to be intimate and talked more openly with her than he had in years. The local cable company rehired him, which was good news. But within two weeks he had slipped back into his old persona—charming but closemouthed, strong but hidden. Soon he was staying out late.

Laurie and Art also suffered a reversal: North Adams was hit with a serious financial setback when its largest employer had a major layoff, and the mini-mall was forced to close.

Art's mother sold the DelNegro sporting-goods shop, leaving Art with no employment; but he secured a good job as manager of the dining facilities at North Adams State College. Laurie spent her time raising the two girls. She talked to her mother daily and visited her father often.

At this time Steven's job ended. He moved in with Art and Laurie and began tending bar. Laurie didn't mind that Steven was staying with them, sleeping on the living-room couch, but his nocturnal hours bothered her, since they didn't coincide with her family's schedule. As her mother had done, Laurie stayed awake late into the night, listening for him to come home.

Laurie wouldn't have minded the imposition or her worrying if Steven were making headway, striving toward something. But he seemed to be doing nothing. Staying at her house was an easy way for him to avoid coming to any decisions. He was, as always, maddeningly casual and unconcerned.

At a party one night, Steven met a man who had been his guidance counselor at Drury High School. The fellow remembered Steven because of his extremely high scores on aptitude and intelligence tests and was surprised that Steven was not on his way to a career. He told Steven that a friend of his, an Air Force recruiter, was looking for young men interested in joining Air Force Intelligence.

Steven's interest was sparked. His father had done intelligence work for the army. He looked up the recruiter, and a week later he took an extensive exam. His scores for aptitude in language and cryptology proved to be the highest first-time results the local administrators had personally seen. The next step—enlistment—was up to Steven, but joining the armed forces was a big commitment. He put off making a decision.

A severe tongue-lashing from Laurie pushed him to enlist. She was tired of worrying about him; she was fed up with tiptoeing around her own house all morning so as not to awaken him; she was done with trying to keep little Kate and Kara quiet for his comfort. She gave him an ultimatum.

"Steven, I love you dearly, but I've had it. Either you do something with your life, or you're going to have to leave."

He left her house and wandered around North Adams for hours. He ended up at the recruiting office near closing time and signed up with the United States Air Force. He stayed with Laurie and Art for another month, until he was sent to Lackland Air Force Base for his basic training.

In 1984 Jean moved out of her apartment on Church Street and moved in with a friend named Jean Todd. Jean Todd and her first husband had been friends of Jean and Manley's years before. Due to turmoil in her own life, Jean Todd had a house all to herself, so she suggested that Jean Tyler move in and share the mortgage payments. Jean agreed with alacrity; it would cost her less than the rent she'd been paying, and she welcomed the company.

The arrangement worked very well. It was good to come home to someone, and the women's friendship deepened. Jean Todd often went with Jean Tyler to visit Manley, as did Angie and Elmer Potter and other friends.

Not long after the relocation, Dr. Joan Hyde phoned with wonderful news.

"Jean, I wanted you to know that Governor Dukakis has commissioned a fact-finding committee on Alzheimer's disease. You've been recommended to sit on the committee."

"What? You've got to be kidding!"

"It's true. Would you be interested?"

"I can't believe you're telling me this. I don't even know what it means."

"It would probably mean a lot of traveling around the state for you, particularly to Boston. There'd be a variety of meetings and hearings and such. But it would be an excellent opportunity to do something for Alzheimer's on a larger scope. It would also mean a lot less free time."

"Free time? What's that?" Jean laughed delightedly. "I'd love to do it if they want me. I'm just not used to this kind of thing."

Jean asked who had recommended her to the governor's committee. Joan professed not to know, but Jean was fairly sure that Joan and Marott Sinex had had something to do with it.

CHAPTER 26

Mid–1984

A few weeks later Jean received a call at home from Governor Michael Dukakis's office. It was official: She was on the Governor's Committee on Alzheimer's Disease. She was stunned. To a humble housewife it seemed unreal, simultaneously exciting and frightening.

She conferred with Joan Hyde and Marott Sinex. They told her that they, too, were on the committee, along with about sixty-five other people of various backgrounds from around the state, including Dr. David Drachman, of the Department of Neurology at the University of Massachusetts. Jay Ellis and he had done research on Alzheimer's disease in the past.

The next time Jean visited Manley, she told him the news.

He smiled in response to her tone of voice and nodded his head.

"Now I'll really be able to do something about Alzheimer's," she said. "You'll see, dear. We'll lick it yet!"

On the way to Boston for the preliminary meetings, Jean was so nervous she almost turned around and went home. But she remembered her cousin Bob MacGowan's words of encouragement when she had voiced her fears to him:

"Don't worry, Jean. You'll do fine. You can accomplish anything."

When she arrived and was being introduced to the people with whom she would be working, she thought, *What in the hell am I doing here? Me. Little Me!*

But she saw that the fancy titles and notoriety of some of the committee members did not make them any more or less human. She gradually relaxed. They were only people, after all.

216

She found herself going to Boston more often and traveling to other parts of the state as well, meeting a host of new people, all with a deep interest and involvement in Alzheimer's disease. The committee's activities, including holding hearings, gathering data, and meeting with groups and organizations across the state, were to span a year. Regular meetings were scheduled so the panel could compare progress, and by year's end the members would submit and publish the results of their fact-finding activities, along with concrete proposals for programs and policy.

At the first meeting the group organized itself into subcommittees. Jean volunteered to serve on the education subcommittee, which was chaired by a sweet man named Tom Goodgame. Jean was chosen to sit in his stead if he was unable to attend meetings. She quickly warmed to her role in the proceedings, and her confidence grew as she saw she could hold her own.

A search was made across the state of Massachusetts for people to testify about every aspect of Alzheimer's disease. There were two hearings: one in Holyoke, to gather testimony from people who lived in the western part of the state, and the other in Boston, for the eastern residents.

The hearing in Boston was held in a large conference room in the State House. It was jammed with people. Every seat was filled, and all standing room was taken. The crowd spilled into the halls and down the stairs.

Like the other committee members, Jean wore a button identifying who she was. She sat among fellow members, reporters, and interested citizens and faced the large curved table where the chairpersons of the various subcommittees flanked Chairman Lewis Weinstein.

The hearing began at nine in the morning and continued nonstop until four in the afternoon. A steady stream of contributors spoke into a microphone at a small table.

Jean listened to professionals and laypersons: family members who were caregivers, nurses, physicians, social workers, lawyers, and community leaders. There were impassioned pleas for financial aid for research. The need to raise community awareness was brought up, as was the necessity for new facilities and programs. There were also harrowing stories of individual experiences with the disease itself, with which Jean was all too familiar.

She was amazed by the extraordinarily intense interest in the disease. She felt heartened that so many other people had been working hard to surmount the public's ignorance about the plight of caregivers.

After the Boston hearing Jean felt much less alone in her struggle. She had not dreamed that so many people were committed to the cause. The scene was similar at the hearing in Holyoke, though slightly less crowded. As far as she knew, Governor Dukakis's committee was the first of its kind, but other states would certainly follow suit.

She had come a long way from the total isolation of her own personal struggle to being a part of a large, organized movement. She hardly had a moment to think these days, though at times it struck her as odd that she hobnobbed with such impressive personages, then returned home to put on her jeans and go back to work at Lamb Printing.

The year's activities were just gearing up. She was asked to appear on a television talk show in Boston called "People Are Talking" on WBZ. For an hour she and three others from the committee discussed Alzheimer's disease and the care of its victims. Jean repeatedly focused attention on the little understood plight of the caregiver.

Later she was invited to participate on radio shows throughout the state, answering questions from people phoning in. She also received invitations to speak to concerned groups and local organizations. This was not the cozy familiarity of groups of people she knew, as her support-group activities had been; she spoke to strangers now, and sometimes the groups were disconcertingly large. But she had a lot to say about Alzheimer's and found she could hold the attention of an audience. After experiencing stage fright many times, she was able to get beyond her nervousness and impart the pertinent information.

Jean and another woman coauthored a proposal for a program to educate nurses, orderlies, and other health-care professionals about Alzheimer's. It was important that the level of care be raised in nursing homes and permanent-care facilities where most workers still knew next to nothing about the disease. They proposed to utilize instructional videotapes and printed literature in ongoing seminars for that purpose.

Jean met with the medical examiner at Berkshire Medical Center and discussed creating a procedure to make it easier for families of deceased Alzheimer's victims to have autopsies done and to donate brain tissue. This was of great importance to reseachers looking for causes and possible treatments.

Jean helped start up yet another Alzheimer's support network, this time centering around the families of patients in the hospital where Manley was placed. Bob Maliken, an energetic hospital social worker, became the facilitator.

Jean made friends with Charlotte Alintuck, the regional representative and vice president of ADRDA. Charlotte also sat on Governor Dukakis's committee. She and Jean agreed there was a need for a separate ADRDA chapter in western Massachusetts.

When Charlotte attended the regular meeting at national headquarters in Chicago, she recommended that a new chapter of ADRDA be started, with Jean Tyler as president. Many months were required for the paperwork and other procedural steps to be completed. Jean, Charlotte Alintuck, Bob Maliken, and a new friend, Wenda Restoff, who ran the Northampton Visiting Nurses Association, drafted a list of people to invite to be board members for the new chapter. The board was formed, and the new western Massachusetts chapter of ADRDA was established, with Jean Tyler as its first president.

CHAPTER 27

1985

*J*ean found satisfaction in working with a legion of like-minded volunteers, battling a common enemy, getting the message out, and planning new strategies. The endless activity kept Jean's mind occupied and was thus a blessing, because Manley slipped evermore from reality.

Jean discovered that men, in general, felt profoundly uncomfortable visiting Manley. Women seemed able to handle the experience better, so his visitors were mainly women. Jean's uncle Teet went for her sake.

Manley's weight had swelled to a thick-waisted one hundred and eighty pounds when he was admitted to the hospital in 1981, since Jean had been feeding him as much as she could; it had been one of his last remaining enjoyments. In the intervening years his weight had steadily declined until, in 1985, he was a gaunt figure of less than a hundred pounds. Uncle Teet and the others found it painful to watch the once robust and bright man wither away.

When Jean came to visit, Manley's face invariably glowed with recognition, and tears were never far behind. He used to say, "Good," when she came, a remnant of "You're so good." Now he was not able to talk at all. His physical coordination had degenerated so profoundly that he had begun to fall. He even needed a restraining chair when sitting so he wouldn't topple out.

He could not feed himself. When Jean was there, she fed him, bringing the spoon to his mouth and wiping his lips of any dribbles.

It was almost impossible to see Manley like this yet still act cheerful. She went less often, occasionally due to her very full schedule but sometimes because she just couldn't bear to see her beloved in this condition. She felt bad if she only saw him once in a week and said so to Head Nurse Ruth Bateman and Natalie, the orderly.

"Manley's sense of time is not tied to reality anymore," Ruth told her. "Regardless of how long it's been since your last visit, to Manley it could seem like five minutes or five years—there's no telling which."

Such mental oblivion was incomprehensible. Jean continued to talk and act with him as if everything was as it used to be. Although he couldn't speak, she told him all about what she had been doing. She operated under the assumption that he might understand some of it.

She tried to act as if things were just fine, keeping her attitude positive and light. After a visit with him she would occasionally feel good, as if communication had passed between them. More often, however, she would be depressed when she left him. The tears blurring her vision made driving home hazardous. She frequently had to pull over and stop the car to let a powerful wave of agony expend itself. Finally, drained of her misery, she could resume her journey home.

Military regimen proved to be good for Steven. For too many years he'd lacked a disciplined framework in his life. Once inside the military's protective system, he blossomed. Now he had the stability of a regulated life; if he followed the rules, everything else was taken care of. He could relax inside his own skin and enjoy being himself.

Once out of boot camp he was sent to the Defense Language Institute in Monterey, California. He was expected to work hard and earn his way through each step. After completing his studies in Monterey he was transferred to another school, in San Angelo, Texas.

There he met Belinda Alamilla, a beautiful nineteen-year-old of Mexican descent. She was studying to be a dental hygienist. The two became inseparable and were married four months later.

Steven brought Belinda home for a visit, and Jean took to her new daughter-in-law. The newlyweds went with Jean to see Manley. Jean was impressed with the way the young bride handled herself.

Belinda went right to the bedside and introduced herself, saying, "Hello, Mr. Tyler, I'm Belinda, Steven's new wife. He's told me so much about you that I feel as if I know you and your family very well. I want you to know that I love Steven very much and will do everything I can to make him happy."

221

Jean thought, *There's a woman after my own heart.*

Steven continued to do well in his studies and was eventually stationed at Howard Air Force Base in Panama, where Belinda and he set up housekeeping. An added bonus of being in the military was that he could play baseball and football. He had found a home.

Manley was unable to eat solid food and, by law, had to be fed liquid nutrients through a tube that went directly into his stomach. Jean resisted any other efforts to keep him alive by machine.

That year her husband had a period of severe agitation, which the nurses and doctors could not understand. He writhed and moaned in distress. A series of X rays revealed that his bowels were blocked, causing his severe pain, and cracking and minute fractures of his vertebrae. The bone was disintegrating, adding to his misery. The staff operated immediately to alleviate the bowel blockage.

Her opinion of the staff caring for her husband rose to open admiration. *Thank God for them,* she thought. *I couldn't find better care for him anywhere.*

After the operation Jean and Laurie were at his bedside as he came out of the anesthesia. When Manley's eyes opened, he raised his head and in a perfectly normal tone said, "Hi."

Jean and Laurie were shocked to the core. He had not spoken a word in over a year. They hugged him and kissed him with joy.

"Daddy," Laurie said, sobbing. "Oh, Daddy! I knew you were all right. I knew it. Everything's going to be all right now! You're going to be well again."

He smiled at his daughter, and then, as clearly as before, he said, "Right."

Those were the last words he ever spoke.

Manley spent weeks in intensive care and was given morphine for the pain from his spine. The drug made him laugh and seem happy much of the time, for which Jean was glad. Anything that was enjoyable to him was welcome. She wanted him to suffer no pain. There was little else anyone could do.

Jean was no longer the shy, tentative public speaker she had been at first. Her passion about the subject of Alzheimer's disease and her natural, down-to-earth humor gave her a lively style. She was asked to speak at an annual governor's conference at the University of Massachusetts in Amherst. The audience she faced filled every seat in the large conference room.

After introducing herself, briefly, describing her experiences with Manley, and discussing some of what she'd learned about

Alzheimer's disease in support groups and committee hearings, Jean said to the audience, "At this moment there are literally millions of people across this country who are spending their life's energy feeding, clothing, washing—doing everything—for a loved one who has Alzheimer's disease. I might as well say they are living for the victim, because their lives are no longer their own. They are victims of Alzheimer's just as surely as the ones they care for, whose brains are being slowly destroyed.

"Alzheimer's changes a victim gradually. Picture the brain as if it were a vast building with a million telephones. The telephones are brain cells, connected to one another. Each day more of them go dead. As seasons pass, there is less of a mind there. The victims are less and less the people they were. It's the growth process in reverse. Slowly the mind regresses until the victim is mentally little more than an infant again. It's not mental retardation or mental illness, although it looks similar at many stages. Those conditions are not fatal and remain relatively stable over the lifetime of a patient and may even improve with treatment. Alzheimer's is progressive and terminal. There's nothing stable about it.

"Watching my father die of leukemia in 1973 was nothing like watching my husband's mind fade away. Right up to the end my father and I could talk. He could tell me what he wanted, and I could help him. He was my dad right up to the end. He knew me, and I knew him. We could communicate.

"An Alzheimer's victim becomes a mere shell of the person he or she was. The body remains, but the mind ever so slowly disappears. It's very strange. You can keep Alzheimer's victims company, and they respond to love, but it reaches a point where they barely know you—if at all. You only have memories of them as they were, because they are radically changed. At rare moments, they may show signs of their old personality, but for the most part, the person that was, is no more.

"My main concern is for the caregivers. They are the forgotten victims of this insidious disease. It's easy to take them for granted—people do it routinely. There's always some good soul in a family willing to do the menial, day-to-day work of taking care of a patient's needs. They are the lowly foot soldiers, the unsung heroes who do the hardest work.

"I ask you not to underestimate what it is they are doing. Believe me, you can't imagine. You can't *know* unless you've been there. With Alzheimer's, the role is unique. The strain is far worse than it would be with an 'ordinary' illness.

"The public's perception of Alzheimer's is that the worst that can happen is the patient becomes forgetful. 'Oh, isn't it a shame, So-and-So can't make coffee anymore.' Believe me, that's the least of it. What really happens is a slow descent into hell.

"One thing that makes it so awful is the time factor. The Alzheimer's victim is going to die, but it will take an average of ten years. *Ten years.* That's a huge chunk out of your life. My husband is still alive, probably because he was unusually young when it started. It's been fourteen years since the onset. He's been hospitalized for almost five of those years."

There were a few gasps from the audience.

Jean nodded knowingly. "The victim, at least, has the blessing of forgetting, but the caregiver is painfully aware every step of the way. As a caregiver you feel the loss not once, not for a few months, but for years. You feel the loss over and over till you think you might go mad. You are literally watching someone's mind die, without the merciful finality of death itself in a reasonable length of time. Alzheimer's drags it out to the limits of human endurance for those who have to watch.

"Death, when it finally comes, is a blessing. Only after the victim's death can a caregiver finally mourn and begin to put his or her life back together—what's left of it," Jean added sarcastically.

"I don't joke lightly about it. Many caregivers never fully recover from the experience. There is a tremendous need for simple understanding by friends and relatives, but because Alzheimer's is so poorly understood by the general public, the caregiver often ends up completely isolated. It's much easier to go through the experience if the burden is shared. But if people don't know the nitty-gritty truth about what caregivers are going through, they can complicate things, confuse issues, make caregivers doubt their own worth. They can—and often do—make a hard situation infinitely worse. And most of it is done with good intentions."

Nervous laughter sounded in the audience.

Jean laughed with them. With an ironic smile, she said, "Caregiving for someone with Alzheimer's is a job for saints—not human beings."

There were a few more uneasy laughs.

Jean put them at ease. "Don't feel embarrassed about laughing. Humor helps. If caregivers can't laugh occasionally, then you know they're in trouble."

She returned to her subject. "Caregivers commonly *downplay* their plight. Remarks such as 'Oh, it's not that bad,' or 'We're getting along fine,' are often a mask. Very often there is a great deal of shame and guilt involved when a family member has a dementing illness.

"I am a proud person. It was not easy for me to admit I needed help. But I sure felt better when I could unburden myself to someone I could trust. Most people, however, couldn't understand. And I couldn't blame them, because so few people know what it's like to care for an Alzheimer's victim. People have to talk more openly about it.

"It's human nature to avoid unpleasant things. People want to think things are 'just fine.' Often, even close relatives won't suspect the true suffering of the caregiver until there's a breakdown in front of them. Can you see how easy it is to lose normal contact with the world? You soon learn to make light of things to spare other people's feelings while you're dying inside. That isolation can destroy lifelong friendships, marriages, and families. It is not uncommon for a caregiver to have a complete emotional breakdown or become seriously ill and even die. You don't know how alone these people can feel."

Jean paused for a long moment to let it sink in. Then she went on, "If people don't know the truth, they can't help. I have seen families in which the father or mother has Alzheimer's, and there are three or four grown children. Typically, only one family member—the spouse or a daughter—will become the primary caregiver. The others may drop by occasionally. Many seem to think that by giving money from time to time, they have discharged their responsibility. Well, money is a big help, but it's not enough. Sometimes other family members will even *criticize* the one doing the caregiving! I'll tell you," her voice rose with understated ferocity, "*that's* grounds for justifiable homicide."

The room erupted in laughter as she smiled impishly.

"Guilt and shame can do a number on you. Caregivers may feel they are somehow to blame. In the later stages of the illness, a caregiver might wish the victim would die, to end everyone's torture. It's healthy to admit those very human feelings. But many people can't handle it. It can ruin their self-worth.

"What I've described to you is not some isolated thing that happens to a rare few. I've seen it over and over in our support meetings. Each day I'm amazed at how pervasive the problem is. There are as many as *four million* cases of Alzheimer's disease in the United States alone.

"I say again: Public ignorance hurts caregivers. That's why I'm here talking about it. Maybe I can make a difference for someone still going through it. Maybe you can pass the word on to others. And if you know someone who is taking care of an Alzheimer's victim, your patience and understanding can help the situation.

"Please learn about it, educate others, and lend your support in any way you can.

"Caregivers need all the help they can get. In a very real way, caregivers become the most needy victims because they live on. They have to continue to face life everyday."

During her speech Governor Michael Dukakis came into the room, listened, then left quietly during the question-and-answer period. Later, during a buffet dinner, Jean was approached by an aide who asked her if she would like to meet the governor.

The room had been so crowded, Jean had not seen Michael Dukakis come in. She followed the aide through the crowd and was introduced to the governor.

"I heard your talk, Mrs. Tyler," he said. "I was very impressed."

Jean found it difficult to make small talk with someone she saw regularly on television. She kept thinking: *Nobody's going to believe this! Little me, talking to the governor!*

She tried to quiet her pounding heart and managed a gracious, "Thank you. I'm so grateful for what you've done, taking the lead in bringing Alzheimer's to the public's attention."

He smiled in appreciation of the compliment. "It's a bigger problem than most of us know, isn't it?"

"Yes," she agreed, gratified that the governor had been affected by her words. "Caregivers need all the help they can get."

"I see that. While listening to you, I realized how much farther we need to go."

As Jean returned to her table, many eyes met hers. She saw herself in their faces. *Caregivers, most of them,* she thought. *Just like me a few years back.*

For a moment she remembered what she had been like in normal times, an unsuspecting and innocent happy housewife. Her ordeal had carried her from an idyllic life through the gates of hell and back. Now she was a savvy organizer-activist, talking to groups like this, listening to a thousand of the saddest stories imaginable, and hearing in each one the echoes of her own tragedy.

She was a changed person. Staring daily into the abyss of horror had changed her, softened her and hardened her all at once. Losing what was most precious to her and being rudely confronted with her all-too-human limitations, she had emerged a very different person from what she could have imagined fifteen years before.

As she sat back in a folding chair and watched another speaker take the lectern, she found herself wanting to share her thoughts with Manley.

A disease has separated us, my love. You are dying slowly in your own personal oblivion. We have no choice but to accept it. I am condemned to live without you. I'm not the bright-eyed Pollyanna I was. But I refuse to be a defeated cynic. I don't know quite who I am anymore, but I think I'm wiser.

Ironically, my life is not so different from what your mission always was: to light the way for those in darkness. It makes me feel useful, helps get me through the day. But I miss you so much.

At least I have the memories of our wonderful life together, of kissing you and feeling your caring arms around me. Your love is still the most solid, comforting thing I've ever known.

Afterword

$\mathcal{M}$anley Tyler died in October 1986. But the death of an Alzheimer's victim rarely ends the suffering of primary caregivers and other loved ones. Such prolonged disruption of life takes its toll. Lowered self-esteem, hopelessness, and guilt linger.

Jean tried not to dwell on the past. Still, there were times when she couldn't help but feel acute loneliness. Since Manley's mind had died so long before, she was surprised to discover that she missed Manley's *physical* presence, even though he'd lain immobile for years in a hospital bed. With his death even that final connection had been severed. Fifteen years of her life, along with the high-school sweetheart who had become her beloved husband had been destroyed by Alzheimer's disease. That chapter was over.

With Manley's death, Jean's monthly disability payments ceased. This made it necessary for her to curtail drastically her networking activities and work primarily to support herself again.

She found herself in financial difficulty because the support network as well as her other volunteerism on behalf of Alzheimer's disease were strictly unpaid. She had donated money to Alzheimer's research and had been so generous in her support work that she had spent thousands of dollars on phone bills, along with other related expenses, quickly dissipating what money she had made from the sale of their home.

Jean's personal growth, becoming a forceful leader and organizer, did not translate into a career in the business world. When she was laboring on behalf of caregivers, she exhibited astonishing drive and confidence. In that selfless cause she was a dynamo of ambition, but it was not in her to use her extensive contacts for personal gain. She was distinctly uncomfortable promoting herself to earn a salary.

AFTERWORD

In 1987 Jean received a Mother's Day card from Steven. It was a huge gag card, measuring more than three feet across and two and a half feet high. He had included a personal note to her, which, after the parent-child problems they had experienced as a result of Manley's disease, were all the more meaningful to her.

He wrote:

It's too bad that only one day a year is alloted to mothers. You are the main link to my success and happiness. You are one of the most well-rounded people I have met or ever care to know. During Dad's illness you were dealing with many variables, unknown and unsuspected factors that would knock most great people to their knees!

A child expects many things from a mother, including love, caring, friendship, a teacher of the necessities, and so on. The child unknowingly receives the ideology of life, what to expect from the world, also discipline and morals.

From a friend you expect advice, love, caring, mutual respect, and mutual interests, ideas or imagination (like yours), in order to enjoy things together.

In a mentor you find character traits to help you gain respect, confidence, and awareness.

Without these three helpers in a person's life, it is very difficult to keep in touch with reality. Without them you would lack support. You would feel very alone. It is possible you could never get in touch with yourself. A person could very easily end up with a past forgotten, an unhappy present, and a very bleak future.

Mom, I think I can speak for Laurie and me in saying we were fortunate enough to have all three and more all rolled up and given to us as our mother.

You could never be completely repaid for all you have done or understand what you have accomplished. But my gratitude grows daily, and I don't know why it takes a Mother's Day for me to let you know.

Love you,

Steven

Life went on. Jean's main joy was her children. To look at Steven one would never know what he'd been through, though Jean knew he must experience his dark moments. Belinda and he lived in Panama till he was transferred to Fort Meade, Maryland, in 1989. He earned continued high praise and advancement and was encouraged to further his education as part of his military commitment. Belinda, meanwhile, finished her studies and became a dental hygienist.

Laurie suffered the worst emotional problems after the death of Manley Tyler. She had always been religious. After her father's death, though, Laurie began to question her faith. She couldn't understand how a merciful God could have allowed such an illness to befall her father, who had always been kind and unselfish. She stopped going to church.

At this same time Laurie suffered a severe case of depression. She had been driving herself mercilessly in her new job as a real-estate saleswoman, while maintaining her duties as wife and mother. One day, for no apparent reason, she could not get out of bed. For a full week she lay in her bedroom, barely eating, refusing even to allow the shades to be lifted to let in sunlight. She experienced headaches, dizziness, and severe neck cramps.

Art took her to visit Dr. Jay Ellis in Pittsfield. The neurologist went to work on her physical symptoms and prescribed a neck brace, massage, and rest. But his understanding of the family situation and his close relationship with the Tylers helped ferret out the underlying cause of Laurie's condition. He spent much time talking to her, more as a friend than as a doctor.

Laurie still felt that she had let her mother and brother down by not being present during the worst of the ordeal with her father. She believed she hadn't suffered enough and abused herself because of it. Jay was of the opinion that she had been overcompensating by overworking herself into emotional and physical exhaustion.

Furthermore, while Jean and Steven had been able to talk out their feelings, Laurie had tried to deny them and suppress them.

Laurie spent many hours talking to Jay, mostly on the phone. He helped her understand that she was as much a victim as Jean and Steven were. Dr. Ellis's help was invaluable, but it was only a beginning.

Free and open discussion with Jean and Steven also helped Laurie. "No one in their right mind *chooses* to go through this kind of experience, Laur," Jean assured her daughter. "When it happens, you do what you have to do because you have no choice. If any of us seems heroic, it's purely against our will."

Laurie had much work to do in the way of introspection, to understand and replace her self-doubt with more positive feelings. It goes on still.

Katie and Kara were asking why they didn't go to church anymore. Art, too, wanted to belong to a church. So after a two-year absence from St. John's Episcopal Church, Laurie met Father Larry Provenzano, who had replaced the retiring Fay Sprague. A cheerful, idealistic young man, he helped Laurie feel good about the Church again. He and his wife became close friends with the Tyler family.

1990

Every Sunday after church Laurie and Art bring the girls to visit their grandmother, and they often eat Sunday dinner together. Jean feels most alive when she is with her children and grandchildren. Their frequent gatherings have the same festive Tyler family atmosphere that existed when Manley was well.

When Belinda and Steven visit, they sleep at Jean's apartment or Laurie and Art's house. Their visits are always charged with high energy, hilarity, and nonstop talk. The family never tires of reliving the good times, of keeping Manley alive in their hearts, of reliving a thousand fond memories.

Steven and Laurie are adamant in their belief that Manley still exists somewhere, somehow. They "talk" to him often, feeling that he is there, watching over them, and occasionally guiding them. They insist that they feel closer to their father after his death than they had for many years of his illness.

Jean doesn't argue with them. For her, Manley is alive in them.

Appendices

Facts on Alzheimer's and Other Dementias

Dementia is the medical term that refers to the loss of intellectual functions such as thinking, remembering, and reasoning, severe enough to impair a person's daily functioning. Symptoms may also include changes in personality, mood, and behavior. Dementia is not itself a disease but a group of symptoms that may accompany certain diseases or conditions. A major difference between dementia and "normal" memory loss is that dementia gets worse with time and affects more than memory.

The most common dementing illness is Alzheimer's disease. Conditions that appear similar to Alzheimer's disease are called *related disorders*. One of the most common related disorders is *multi-infarct dementia*. This condition is caused by multiple strokes (infarcts) in the brain. Alzheimer's disease and multi-infarct dementia occur together in fifteen to twenty percent of dementia patients.

Some of the other well-known diseases that produce dementia include: Parkinson's disease, Huntington's disease, Pick's disease, Creutzfeldt-Jakob disease, amyotrophic lateral sclerosis (Lou Gehrig's disease), and multiple sclerosis. Other conditions that can cause or mimic dementia include: normal pressure hydrocephalus, depression, brain tumors, thyroid disorders, blood chemistry imbalances, nutritional and vitamin deficiencies, alcoholism, infections (meningitis, syphilis, AIDS), head injuries, and drug intoxication and interaction. Some of these conditions may be reversible or treatable.

Alzheimer's is noted by physical damage to brain tissue in the form of microscopic structural abnormalities called *senile plaques* and *neurofibrillary tangles,* whose causes are unknown. These structures occur in normal brain tissue but in far smaller quantities.

The disease is also characterized by a lack of chemical (neurotransmitter) acetylcholine, and somatostatin, needed for messages to pass from one brain cell (neuron) to another.

Alzheimer's disease is irreversible. Medical research has so far failed to find a cause or cure for it. At present there is no known treatment to slow or stop its progress. It is also called Alzheimer's Dementia or Senile Dementia of the Alzheimer's Type (SDAT). It was first described by German physician Alois Alzheimer in 1907, when it was considered a rare disorder. It knows no social or economic boundaries and affects men and women almost equally. By conservative estimates it now claims 4.5 million victims in the United States and impacts on the lives of a far greater number of people, particularly those who devote time and energy every day to care for the victims.

Most research indicates that about fifty percent of all cases of dementia are caused by Alzheimer's, twenty percent are caused by multi-infarct disease (stroke), and another twenty percent are caused by a combination of the two. The remaining ten percent are due to one of the many other causes.

It is more likely to occur as a person gets older. After age sixty-five, as many as ten percent of people may develop Alzheimer's, and over age eighty-five the figure may reach as high as forty-seven percent. The youngest documented case of Alzheimer's disease is that of a twenty-eight year old.

Symptoms

The onset of Alzheimer's is usually gradual. Victims exhibit slow decline in many areas of intellectual ability, accompanied by physical decline in later stages. Early on, memory may seem to be the only area affected (particularly memory of recent events). A decline in the ability to perform routine tasks is likely, as well as disorientation and confusion. Depression may occur, along with noticeable personality changes. Difficulty in abstract thinking and learning is not unusual. The victims may have trouble at work and may not enjoy reading as much as before. Language and motor skills deteriorate. Handwriting may change. When talking, they may have difficulty choosing the correct words, finishing thoughts, or following directions. There may be uncharacteristic outbursts of anger and even violence. Victims seem to become more childlike, with a loss of judgment and comprehension of even simple matters. A tendency for wandering aimlessly is common.

With time there may be a noticeable stoop or shuffle in the victim's walk. Late in the illness the victims become severely impaired, incontinent, and even unable to walk. They may invent words and later be unable to speak at all. They may not be able to recognize anyone or just one or two loved ones. The rate of deterioration varies from person to person, but at some point they become totally unable to care for themselves. By then they will need nursing care and must be constantly monitored.

Alzheimer's disease eventually leaves the victim physically less resistant to infections such as pneumonia. This is a common cause of death in such cases. The older population that it affects is subject to other chronic illnesses, which may also be the cause of death. Death may occur in as few as three or four years or may take as long as fifteen years.

Diagnosing Alzheimer's Disease

There is no single diagnostic test for Alzheimer's disease. At present, diagnosis can only be done by eliminating all other causes of the person's symptoms. Complete physical, psychiatric, and neurologic evaluation is necessary. A complete diagnostic workup includes the following:

- *Detailed Patient History.* The patient's medications, behavior, and past medical problems must be evaluated. No detail is too trivial to be of importance.
- *Complete Physical and Neurological Examinations.*
- *Mental Status Exam and Neuropsychological Testing.*
  These tests can help in diagnosing depression, which can cause confusion and memory loss in older people.
- *Laboratory Tests.* Blood work, urinalysis, chest X ray, electroencephalography (EEG), and electrocardiogram (EKG).
- *Brain Scans.* CT scan (or CAT scan), PETT scan, and MRI scan. These do not diagnose Alzheimer's disease but assist in eliminating other treatable diseases or disorders.

The accuracy of such diagnosis by elimination is about ninety percent. An absolute diagnosis of the disease can only be made by studying the brain tissue under a microscope, usually at autopsy, to discover the presence of tangles of fibers (neurofibrillary tangles) and clusters of degenerating nerve endings (senile plaques) in areas of the brain important for memory and intellectual functions.

236

Normal Memory Loss

As they get older many healthy individuals are less able to remember certain types of information. Health-care professionals use the term "age-associated memory impairment" (AAMI) to describe minor memory difficulties that come with age.

AAMI is not disabling or progressive. Dementias are both. AAMI is often most noticeable when an individual is under pressure. Once the person has relaxed again, he or she is able to remember forgotten material without difficulty.

Besides memory impairment due to age, minor memory difficulties may be caused by distraction, fatigue, grief, depression, stress, illness, medication, alcohol or other drugs, vision or hearing loss, lack of concentration, or an attempt to remember too many details at once.

Whereas dementia is progressive, AAMI may remain unchanged for years. Most people with AAMI can compensate for memory loss with reminders and notes. Dementia, on the other hand, will eventually interfere with normal activities of daily life.

Research into Causes

Efforts to find a cause and cure for Alzheimer's disease are complicated by indications that there may be more than one form of the disease.

Neuropathology (the study of the diseased nervous system)

Much information has been gained through autopsies on the brains of deceased Alzheimer's victims. Most notable discoveries are the formations of senile plaques and neurofibrillary tangles, which occur in previously healthy nerve cells. In addition, scientists have found Alzheimer brains to contain *amyloids,* small protein fragments, located in the blood vessels and in the cores of plaques. Alzheimer brains also show shrinkage or atrophy.

Biochemistry (the study of chemical processes in living beings)

Researchers have found abnormally low amounts of some message-carrying chemicals (neurotransmitters) in the brain of Alzheimer's victims. The most studied neurotransmitter, acetylcholine (ACH), has been found to be deficient in the same areas of the brain where plaques and tangles are found. Parkinson's disease is noted by a deficiency of the neurotransmitter dopamine. A drug, L-Dopa, has been developed that now can be taken to alleviate Parkinson's symptoms.

There is also research into toxins (poisons) and their possible relationship to the disease. Most of this research has centered on the presence of increased amounts of aluminum in Alzheimer's brains. It is not known if this is a cause or result, however.

Virology (the study of viruses)

Viruses are being studied to see if the disease could be due to a slow spreading virus in the brain, as is the cause with Creutzfeldt-Jakob disease, which exhibits symptoms similar to Alzheimer's disease. The body's immune system is the focus of some studies to see if aberrations in the system could be a cause.

Genetics (the study of genes)

Considerable research has gone into possible hereditary causes of Alzheimer's disease. The most active area of this effort is on chromosome 21 of the DNA molecule. Some scientists believe that this may be a promising area of research because of the relationship between Alzheimer's and Down's syndrome. Down's syndrome (mongolism) results in mental retardation and other birth defects. People with Down's syndrome have an extra chromosome 21.

Individuals with Down's syndrome who survive into middle age frequently develop changes in the brain that are identical to an Alzheimer's brain. Additionally, chromosome 21 contains the gene that manufactures amyloid (protein fragments), which are found in plaques and blood vessels of brain tissue of Alzheimer's victims.

A new tool called *positron emission transaxial tomography* (PETT) enables scientists to see just what parts of the brain become active when the brain does specific things. Using this to compare sick and normal brain activity could lead to clues about Alzheimer's disease in the future.

Blood flow and nutrition are being studied for clues to cause or treatment. New drugs also continue to be tested.

Caregiver's Needs

Caregivers are also casualties of Alzheimer's. Since there is no known cure or treatment, we can do little for the victims except to provide love and gentle care to minimize emotional and physical suffering. But those who care for them day by day may suffer as much or more; we can only estimate the number of families and individuals whose existence has been ruined as a side effect of this illness. The emotional turmoil often continues after the victim's death. Caregivers who watch lifelong bonds of communication disappear due to a loved one's brain dysfunction can suffer self-doubt, guilt, and intense loneliness from which many can't recover without guidance and support from those experienced in this very specific problem.

Millions of family members and caregivers desperately need help in dealing with the heartbreak of watching a victim's mind die. The practical, social, legal, and psychological problems are complex and unique and are exacerbated by public ignorance of what these caregivers have to deal with.

If you are a caregiver for a dementia victim, here are some suggestions to help you care for yourself:

Ask for help.

No one will know what you're going through unless you tell them. Outsiders often need some direction from you on how they can help with your daily duties, household chores, or errands. Try not to rely on only one source of support. Communicate your needs, fears, and problems as well as your gratitude.

Take care of your health.

Exercise! Try to maintain the same exercise activities you had before you became a caregiver.

Ask a friend, neighbor, or family member to stay with the victim while you go for a walk or enjoy some other form of beneficial vigorous activity.

Keep your own appointments with physicians, dentists, counselors, etc.

Rest when the victim rests, or do something special for yourself.

Get out of the house for a period of time each day.

Have someone who is willing to take care of the victim sleep over occasionally so you can get an uninterrupted night's sleep.

Try to maintain your outside interests and activities.

Don't lose your sense of humor.

If you have an opportunity to laugh, do it. Find ways to enjoy each day.

Try to avoid feeling guilty.

Remember that you have nothing to do with your loved one's rate of deterioration.

Pace yourself.

Do what is most important, then do more only if you have the energy. If you're tired, stop.

Know yourself.

Know when the stresses are becoming too much to bear and what you need to do to regain your strength and objectivity. Don't feel that you have to do everything yourself. Forgive yourself if things don't go just right.

Give yourself credit for a job well done.

Remind yourself of the value of what you're doing. It's hard to imagine a more difficult job.

Counseling.

Psychotherapy for family members, including spouses, children, grandchildren, and, of course, the primary caregiver can help by drawing everyone into a cooperative effort. Each person has his own point of view and mutual examination of the goals and realities can bring people closer together, making things easier on everyone.

Don't isolate yourself.

Keep in touch with friends. You may have to initiate contact. People may hesitate to call, not wanting to intrude or interrupt at a bad time.

Allow time for your feelings.

Find someone you can talk to. Attend a support-group meeting where you can express your feelings.

Support groups:

You might be surprised at the value of what you can learn by talking to others in similar straits. A support network can give you the opportunity to:

~ be listened to

~ obtain practical information from others

~ learn about community services

~ receive love and moral support from other caregivers

It is common for family members and caregivers to feel isolation, anger, helplessness, resentment, embarrassment, grief, guilt, jealousy, frustration, fear, and panic. A support group is a place where you can express your concerns and feelings with others who are experiencing the same emotions.

Attend a support group that meets your needs. There are many different types, from small, intimate groups to larger, more formal gatherings with speakers and presentations. You may need a group geared for people currently giving care or a group for those whose loved one has already passed on. The problems associated with the stress of caregiving do not necessarily go away after the victim has died.

Call Alzheimer's Association (formerly ADRDA) for a list of support groups in your area. It is a rich resource of guidance for a variety of issues, including sources of help in financial and legal matters. Alzheimer's Association was formed by people experienced with Alzheimer's disease and whose goal it is to help the growing number of caregivers. The toll-free phone number where they can be reached is:

1-800-621-0379 (In Illinois: 1-800-572-6037)

The address for national headquarters is:

ALZHEIMER'S ASSOCIATION
70 East Lake Street
Chicago, IL 60601-5997

Planning Ahead

As dementia progresses, financial and legal matters will be affected. At some point a family member or other concerned individual will need to assume responsibility for decision making. Failure to prepare could be devastating. The following suggestions and guidelines may be of help.

Legal considerations:

Learn about durable power of attorney, conservatorship, guardianship, living trust, living will, and other legal options. Consult with an adviser who is experienced with the legal and financial affairs of older persons or contact Alzheimer's Association. It exists to help people who are dealing with Alzheimer's.

The Legal Aid Society or the local Office on Aging can help you find legal aid that is free or offered at a low cost. Many bar associations provide free or reduced-fee legal advice for those who need it. Other sources of affordable legal help are law-school programs or local legal clinics.

Laws vary from state to state. Find out what the legal specifics are in your area.

Get a valid signature on legal documents while the victim is still able and competent to sign.

Locate insurance policies, wills, bankbooks, automobile titles, tax records, safe-deposit-box keys, etc.

Support-group members and other families who have dealt with some of the practical problems you now face are excellent sources of information. Ask them about their experiences.

Financial considerations:

The finances of families of Alzheimer's victims can be devastated over the prolonged time—usually seven to ten years—the disease usually lasts. Costs will probably include: lost income (since the victim will be unable to work), transportation costs, medical care, respite services, and nursing-home care. Planning is imperative.

The loss of independence and "power of the purse" can exacerbate the suspicions and resentment an Alzheimer's victim feels toward others. Delusions of "someone stealing from me" or "trying to trick me" are common with Alzheimer's disease, even though the person may not have been prone to suspicion before. It is the nature of the disease and must be expected.

Making the necessary legal changes to safeguard family finances can be very difficult if the victim resists. You may need support from relatives, friends, professionals, or clergy.

Medicare and most private health-insurance programs do not pay for services provided in the home or in a nursing home. Only Medicaid and a few private insurance policies pay for nursing-home care. Medicaid regulations are complex and change often. Seek knowledgeable help and advice from Alzheimer's Association, a support group, or a lawyer or financial adviser who knows about Medicaid regulations.

Financial assistance can be sought in several areas, including government entitlement programs. Entitlement programs cover two general areas of assistance for Alzheimer's victims: those that supplement income for the patient and/or dependent family members, and those that help pay medical expenses.

Financial Support Programs

Social Security Disability assists wage earners under the age of sixty-five who can no longer work because of a disability. An applicant must have worked at least five out of the previous ten years, though they need not be in consecutive years.

To apply for Social Security Disability, contact your local Social Security office listed under "Social Security Administration" in the phone book.

Supplemental Security Income (SSI) provides monthly income to the aged, disabled, and blind who have limited income and assets. If the victim is over sixty-five you may obtain higher benefits by qualifying as an "aged" person rather than disabled.

To apply for SSI, contact your local Social Security office.

Aid to Families with Dependent Children (AFDC) offers financial assistance for youngsters whose parents cannot support them. Benefits also support the parents or adults who care for the children. The requirements for AFDC are strict, but the family, once eligible, also qualifies for Medicaid. Contact the local office of your state welfare agency to apply for AFDC.

Medical Expense Programs

Medicare is federal health insurance, usually for people over age sixty-five who receive Social Security retirement benefits. Though its medical coverage can be very helpful, it does not cover all the needs of the Alzheimer's victim. Contact your local Social Security office to apply.

Medicaid is federally funded but varies from state to state. Not all facilities accept Medicaid. Contact your local welfare agency to apply for Medicaid.

Older Americans Act helps people over age sixty. To apply, contact your state department on aging.

Social Services Block Grant assists low-income children and adults. To apply, contact your state department of social services.

To protect your rights:

- You may need to talk to a lawyer about how the assets are divided among the family.
- It is important to document everything. Make copies of every form you fill out and every letter you write. On the phone, ask for the names of people you talk to and make dated notes of the conversations. Having such notes and copies will assist in appealing applications for financial assistance.
- Keep all receipts and tax records. Make sure you have current copies of insurance policies and employee benefits. You can obtain a Disability Documentation Kit from the Alzheimer's Association chapter near you to help with your record keeping.
- Be persistent in dealing with government agencies. Many applications are approved after being rejected the first time. Don't give up.
- Alzheimer's Association can refer you to other sources of information and assistance.

Tips for the Caregiver

Communicating with the Alzheimer's Patient

- Give one direction or ask one question at a time.
- When speaking with the patient, be calm and reassuring. Speak slowly and distinctly, using simple words and short sentences.
- It is helpful to be a good listener. Your genuine interest conveys respect and concern.
- Smile, nod, touch, and make eye contact. Your tone of voice and body language are as important as words.
- Avoid slang or idioms that can cause confusion if taken literally, such as "take a hike" or "you're pulling my leg."
- Ask questions that require only one choice at a time: for example, "Do you want coffee?" instead of "Do you want coffee or tea?"
- Use humor but do not laugh at a victim's inappropriate speech.
- Dementia patients may be able to understand more than they can express. Remember that this can lead to frustration because they are unable to make themselves understood.
- Be sensitive to the fact that dementia patients still hear and may understand what is being said about them. Don't talk to others about the patient as if he or she were not there.

Dealing with Memory Loss

- Establish a simple, consistent daily routine and adhere to it as much as possible.
- The patient's ability to remember will vary from day to day and will gradually decrease over time. Your expectations may need to change as well.

- Keep regularly used items in their usual place so they can be easily located.
- Recognition is easier than recall. "Here is your granddaughter Mary" is more helpful than "Do you remember who this is?"
- As long as the patient continues to understand written words, signs and labels can be useful reminders of what items are and how they are used. Label household goods and rooms with words or pictures.
- Digital clocks may be easier to read than conventional ones.
- Display a bulletin board with a day, date, and season printed clearly.
- Display pictures of friends and family with their names written underneath.

Depression

Many Alzheimer's victims are understandably depressed, especially in the early stages. They feel a loss. They have become more dependent and might have feelings of failure. The depression is treatable, even if the illness is not. Reassurance will help.

Some common signs of depression are withdrawal, reduced concentration, hopelessness, restlessness, loss of appetite, early rising, and poor sleeping or over-sleeping during the day.

- Encourage exercise. Alcohol should be avoided.
- Avoid giving false hope or patronizing "pep talks."
- Encourage the patient to talk about or express his or her feelings.
- Notice whether certain activities or people trigger moments of depression or an improvement in mood. Build upon the activities that create positive results and try to minimize the others.
- Don't force the patient to socialize but encourage him or her to be as socially active as possible.

Wandering

Wandering can be dangerous for the person with Alzheimer's. Wanderers may not realize they are lost. They may walk into dangerous situations and become traffic or crime victims. They are also at risk of exposure and exhaustion.

It is helpful if the patient carries some form of identification, such as a necklace, bracelet, or wallet card containing name, address, phone number, medical data, and the information that the person is memory impaired.

Give the name and description of the patient, with a recent photograph, to local police and fire departments.

Hostile and Demanding Behavior

Alzheimer's may create unpleasant and inappropriate behavior in the victim.

- Irritability and belligerence can be a sign of physical pain. Ask the victim directly if he or she is in pain.

- Belligerence may also mean he feels badly about himself. A warm, nonjudgmental approach including simple courtesies such as saying "please" and "thank you" indicate that you accept him as he is.

- Try not to show your anger. The patient's annoying behavior is usually not intentional. The victim may not remember what is expected.

- Saying no calmly and firmly, then redirecting the person's attention, may defuse a tense situation.

- Sometimes merely ignoring demands will work.

- Alzheimer's victims become childlike as the disease progresses. A doll or stuffed animal may have a calming, soothing effect.

- Pets seem to have a calming effect on dementia patients. If keeping a dog or cat is not feasible, try animals that don't require as much care, such as birds or fish.

Catastrophic Reactions

Sometimes a dementia victim will have a reaction out of proportion to events because of confusion or overstimulation. Unfamiliar places, loud noises, new people, and uncertainty about a task can provoke excessive emotions such as weeping, shouting, or striking out.

- Plan activities to minimize the aforementioned situations. Reduce confusion in the patient's environment. Remove him or her from a distressing situation and cautiously distract attention with an activity the patient can easily do and enjoy.

- If a task is becoming too difficult, simplify it or redirect the patient to another activity.

247

- Do not ask an agitated patient to make a decision.
- Restrain physically only if absolutely necessary.

Hallucinations and Delusions

Victims of Alzheimer's disease sometimes see or hear things that are not there (hallucinations) or believe things that are not true (delusions).

- Medications or other illnesses can be a cause. A physician should be consulted.
- Whispering or laughing in front of an Alzheimer's patient may be misinterpreted.
- If the person appears to be hallucinating, leave him or her alone or approach slowly to avoid causing fear.
- False accusations may result from deluded thinking or may simply be a way of looking for reassurance. For instance, a woman who accuses her husband of infidelity may only want to be reassured that her husband won't leave her.
- Try to interpret what the experience means to the deluded or hallucinating person or respond to the emotion being expressed. For example, "Do you think someone stole your money?" or "It sounds as if you are frightened."
- Avoid arguing or trying to explain that what the patient is thinking, seeing, or hearing is not real. It is real to the victim.

Sexuality

Sexually oriented behavior can be embarrassing and difficult to manage with the dementia victim. Discussing it with friends and family can also be a problem.

- Indiscreet fondling of himself, touching others, and suggestive fidgeting should be gently discouraged. Try redirecting his attention.
- If a patient exposes himself, he may need to use the bathroom. If he disrobes, he may want to go to bed.

Household Safety

- Have working fire extinguishers and smoke alarms.
- Keep a list of emergency numbers by every phone.
- Keep walkways clear. Avoid scatter rugs and exposed extension cords. Consider removing small pieces of furniture.

- Poisons, chemicals, and medications should be locked away or kept out of reach.
- Remove firearms or keep them locked up.
- Removing the knobs from the stove and disconnecting appliances can prevent a kitchen fire. Or you may restrict access to the kitchen. You may also shut off the circuit or loosen a fuse when appliances are not in use.
- Avoid look-alike objects such as fruit-shaped magnets on refrigerator.
- Hide a spare key outside the house in case the patient locks you out.
- Consider painting the top and bottom stairs a different color from the others.
- Keep attic and basement doors locked.
- Use safety locks on windows.
- Provide good lighting throughout the house.
- Remove all poisonous plants, such as coleus, philodendron, and poinsettia.

Sources of Help

Alzheimer's Association (formerly ADRDA, Alzheimer's Disease
and Related Disorders Association) is a nonprofit organization
founded in 1980. It provides information and support to families,
public education about Alzheimer's disease and other dementing
illnesses, and support for research.

It now has over 190 chapters throughout the U.S. Each chapter
sponsors multiple support groups and affiliates. You can call
Alzheimer's Association for information on patient management
and community resources, for a list of support groups and special-
ized diagnostic clinics in your area, for information about the legal
and financial problems faced by care givers, or just to talk to a sympathetic listener. Again the phone numbers:

The toll-free phone number is: 1-800-621-0379

In Illinois: 1-800-572-6037 or 1-312-853-3060

The address for the national headquarters is:

ALZHEIMER'S ASSOCIATION
70 East Lake Street
Chicago, IL 60601-5997

Home Care Corporations arrange for help with housework,
transportation, and meals and can also provide respite (relief) for
the care giver. They are a good place to call for information about
community services.

Other sources of help include:

Councils on Aging

Visiting Nurses Associations

Home Health Agencies
Adult Day Programs
Private Geriatric Care Managers
Elder Legal Services
Social Security Administration
Department of Public Welfare
Veterans Administration
Hospital Social Workers

Counseling Services
Family Service Agencies
Mental Health Clinics
Pastoral Counselors
Private Therapists

Further Reading

Financial

Your Right to Appeal Your Medical Insurance Payment
Available from Department of Health and Human Services, Health Care Financing Administration, 200 Independence Ave., S.W., Washington, DC 20201

Your Medicare Handbook
Available through your local Social Security office.

Medicaid/Medicare: Which is Which?
Available from the Department of Health and Human Services.

Losing a Million Minds (Chapter 11)
Congressional Office of Technology Assessment.
Philadelphia, PA: J.B. Lippincott, 1987.

Disability Documentation Kit
Available from Alzheimer's Association.

General

Understanding Alzheimer's Disease
by Miriam K. Aronson, Ed.D. (ed.).
N.Y.: Scribners, Summer, 1988.

The Loss of Self: A Family Resource for the Care of Alzheimer's Disease and Related Disorders
by Donna Cohen, Ph.D., and Carl Eisdorfer, Ph.D., M.D.
N.Y.: W.W. Norton & Co., 1986.

FURTHER READING

The 36-Hour Day: A Family Guide to Caring for Persons with Alzheimer's Disease and Related Dementing Illnesses
by Nancy L. Mace and Peter V. Rabins, M.D.
Baltimore: Johns Hopkins University Press, 1981.*

Dementia: A Practical Guide to Alzheimer's Disease and Related Illnesses
by Leonard L. Heston, M.D., and June A. White.
N.Y.: W.H. Freeman, 1983.*

Alzheimer's Disease: The Silent Epidemic
by Julia Frank, M.D.
Minneapolis: Lerner Publications Company, 1985.

Much of the information in this appendix was obtained from: *Alzheimer's Disease and Related Disorders Family Care Guide* by the eastern Massachusetts Chapter of ADRDA (Alzheimer's Disease and Related Disorders Association, Inc.) in collaboration with the Chapters of western Massachusetts and Cape Cod and the Islands, 1988, and assorted pamphlets of ADRDA.

---

* Available from the Alzheimer's Association national headquarters and chapters.